English for Pharmaceutical Sciences

入門薬学英語

CD付き

野口ジュディー
神前陽子
籠田智美
山口秀明

講談社サイエンティフィク

まえがき

　本書は，薬学分野の専門英語に的をしぼり，薬学部の大学学部生を対象として編集された英語の教科書です．薬学専攻の学生として，この教科書を手にしたみなさんには，まず原点に帰って，「なぜ，大学で英語を勉強するのか？」という問いを自らに向かって投げかけてほしいと思います．教養のため？それとも，ただ，単にカリキュラムに組み込まれているから？英語が好きだからという人もいるでしょう（もちろん，それ自体は素晴らしいことです！）

　答えは，実は，みなさんの中というよりは，むしろ，薬学専攻の学生としてのみなさんを取り巻く社会状況の中にあります．医薬品は国際商品で，その開発も情報の蓄積も国際的な連携の中で同時に進行しています．インターネットなどの急速な発展が，この状況にさらに拍車をかけています．臨床適用や薬品の主作用，副作用データなど，必要な情報を得ようと思えば，好むと好まざるに関わらず英語で発信された情報を読まなければなりません．

　では，実際に，薬学業務に携わるうちに，英語で書かれた文書に取り組まざるをえなくなったときの状況を想像してみてください．取り組むべき文書は，一般の教科書のように，英語を母国語としない人のために平易に書き下ろしたものでしょうか？これも，答えははっきりしています．みなさんが，卒業後，取り組む文書は，すべて，語学学習用ではなく，本来の目的のために書かれたものです．そして，読者も英語という言語に不自由を感じていない人たちを対象としています．当然のことながら，これらの文書は，みなさんには，一見，難しく手ごわく見えることでしょう．

　しかし，困難なことばかりではありません．みなさんが，これまで取り組んできた受験英語とは異なり，これら「本物」の文書にはタイトルがあり，情報源，著者名，出版社名などが通常記されています．また，文書のレイアウトや，一見して見てとれる文体の特徴などは，新聞記事には新聞記事の，学術論文には学術論文の，薬品の効能書には薬品の効能書のというように，そのジャンルに特有の視覚的情報を提供しており，「この文書が，一体，何なのか？」を一目で特定する助けとして機能しています．これらの情報を手がかりに，文書の「目的」，対象としている「読者」，盛り込まれているであろう「情報」

を予測するならば,手ごわく見える文書も,今持っている英語力でなんとか扱えるのではないか——という考えのもとに,この教科書は作られています.そして,文書が何の目的(purpose)で,誰を読者(audience)として想定して書かれたものかを考え,伝えるべき情報(information)を最も効率よく伝達するのに,言語がどのように使われているか,その特徴(language features)を観察することによって,学習者が「この文書が専門分野でどのような働きをもっているのか」という洞察に達することを最終目標としています.

　上記のような理由から,この教科書では,実際に世の中に出回っているさまざまな「ジャンルの文書」を学習者用に加工せずに提示しています.そして何よりもこれらの文書は,みなさんが卒業後,薬学業務に携わる際に出会うであろう文書という基準に沿って,薬学の分野の専門家に集めてもらったものです.練習問題は,文書から情報を探して取り出すという,「読む」という本来の作業プロセスをシミュレートするようにデザインされています.また,図や表からできるだけ情報を得る練習や,段落ごとに最初の文のみを拾い読みする練習は,情報をできるだけ早く正確に得ることを目的としています.そして,せっかく得た情報は,必要に応じて自由に取り出せるよう,保持されなければなりません.そのために情報を分類,整理するテクニックも数多く提案しています.

　みなさんには,この教科書が提案しているアプローチを,最初は非常に意識的に用い,次には習慣として定着させてほしいと思います.すなわち,言語の特徴を観察(Observe)して),観察したことを整理し(Classify),使い方を色々考えてみて(Hypothesize),考えたことを実際に試してみる(Apply)というプロセスの繰り返しです.この教科書で学ぶことが,卒業後の生涯学習としての英語学習に正しい方向性を与え,やがて,みなさんが薬学の専門家として必要な国際語としての英語をしっかり身につけ,その使い手に成長していくことを願ってやみません.

2007年　晩冬

著者一同

contents

Preface ii

Unit 1 *Safety advice*
SunWise Program 1
(Environmental Protection Agency, USA)

Unit 2 *Advice column*
Red wine good, red wine bad: which advice should I believe? 6
(The Times, UK)

Unit 3 *Public health notification*
Contact lenses and eye infections 12
(Food and Drug Administration, USA)

Unit 4 *Wiki*
Headache 20
(Wikipedia, Internet)

Unit 5 *Public announcement*
Collection of syringes by pharmacies 26
(Environmental Bureau of the Tokyo Metropolitan Government, Japan)

Unit 6 *Public information from professional organization*
Food Allergies and Reactions 35
(American Academy of Allergy Asthma and Immunology, USA)

Unit 7 *News article*
Childhood deaths in Japan bring new look at flu drug 42
(New York Times)

目次

前書き　ii

Unit1　安全に関する勧告
対紫外線安全策　1
（環境保護庁，アメリカ）

Unit2　助言コラム
赤ワインを飲むべきか？
飲まざるべきか？　6
（The Times，イギリス）

Unit3　健康に関する公式通知
コンタクトレンズと眼感染症　12
（食品医薬品局，アメリカ）

Unit4　ウィキー
頭痛　20
（ウィキペディア，インターネット）

Unit5　公告
薬局による使用済み注射針の回収　26
（東京都環境局，日本）

Unit6　専門家の機関からの情報
食品アレルギーとアレルギー反応　35
（米国アレルギー・喘息・免疫学会，アメリカ）

Unit7　新聞記事
日本における小児の死亡がもたらす
抗インフルエンザ薬への新たな見解　42
（New York Times，アメリカ）

v

Unit8 `Fact sheeat`
Fact sheet on avian flu 50
(Centers for Disease Control and Prevention, USA)

Unit9 `Government report`
National Report on Human Exposure to Environmental Chemicals 56
(Centers for Disease Control and Prevention, USA)

Unit10 `Textbook`
Cardiovascular system: scheme of blood circulation 65
(The Anatomy Coloring Book, UK)

Unit11 `Patient information sheet`
What is metabolic syndrome? 71
(American Heart Association, USA)

Unit12 `Textbook`
Lipid-lowering drugs and atherosclerosis: Therapeutic overview 78
(Human Pharmacology, USA)

Unit13 `Patient information sheet`
On therapy for diabetes mellitus 88
(American Diabetes Association, USA)

Answers to "英語あれこれノート" 99

Understanding pharmacy terms with affixes 101

Vocabulary Index 111

Unit8　事実記録
鳥インフルエンザに関する重要な事実　　50
（疾病管理予防センター，アメリカ）

Unit9　政府公告
環境化学物質曝露に関する国の報告　　56
（疾病管理予防センター，アメリカ）

Unit10　教科書
循環器系：血液循環の模式図　　65
（The Anatomy Coloring Book，イギリス）

Unit11　患者用の情報
メタボリックシンドローム（代謝症候群）
とは何か？　　71
（米国心臓協会，アメリカ）

Unit12　教科書
高脂血症治療薬と動脈硬化：
治療の概要　　78
（Human Pharmacology，アメリカ）

Unit13　勧告
糖尿病における栄養療法　　88
（米国糖尿病学会，アメリカ）

英語あれこれノート　解答　　99

接頭辞・接尾辞でみる薬学用語　　101

用語索引　　111

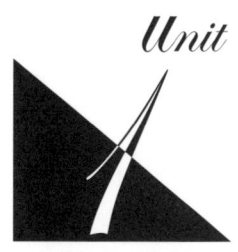

Genre: **Safety advice**

Source: **United States Environmental Protection Agency**

EPA（Environmental Protection Agency） 米国環境保護庁

　アメリカ合衆国の環境政策全般を担当する行政組織で，日本の環境省に相当する．本部はワシントンD.C. にあり，10ヶ所の地方支部局および10数カ所の研究所が設置され，全国に約18,000人の職員を擁する．人の健康，大気・水質・土壌などの環境保護・保全を組織のミッション（目標）と位置づけており，(1) 大気汚染，水質汚濁，残留農薬等による食糧汚染，(2) 有害化学物質による環境汚染，廃棄物処理や管理に伴う汚染拡散の防止・対策，(3) 地球規模の環境問題のリスク削減等に関する規制措置，(4) 環境情報の整備や環境教育の支援等を通じて，住民の参加や意思決定の材料等を提供している．上位機関として，大統領直属の環境諮問委員会（**CEQ**）があり，大統領の意向に基づき各省庁の連携・調整を図っている．なお，自然環境行政に関しては，日本では，環境省内の自然環境局が担当しているが，米国においては，主に内務省の国立公園局および魚類・野生生物局が担当している．

SunWise Program　URL▸▸▸ http://www.epa.gov/sunwise/

　EPAによる紫外線対策のプログラム．米国では，国民の5人に1人が皮膚癌になるといわれており，深刻な問題になっている．そのため，全国の学校・地域社会を通して，国民に太陽と安全に付き合うための教育を行っている．初等教育における活動が活発で，小学生や保護者向けに，(1) 各地域における紫外線指数の測定・公表，(2) 成層圏のオゾン層破壊・紫外線に関する教育，(3) 日常生活における紫外線対策教育，(4) 専門家による講演等を行っている．

Observing the text as a whole

　Look at the following page and think about its PAIL characteristics. （**PAIL**: **P** = Purpose　文章の目的, **A** = Audience　文章の対象者, **I** = Information　情報の内容, **L** = Language features　文章の構成形態）

Genre:	Advice　アドバイス
Purpose:	To provide advice about protection from overexposure to ultraviolet rays from the sun　紫外線への過剰曝露を防ぐためのアドバイス
Audience:	General public　一般の人々
Information:	Sun safety　対紫外線安全策
Language features:	Imperative verbs for each action　対策ごとに命令文を使用
	Complete sentences for explanations　文法上省略を含まないセンテンス
	Pictures to represent each action step　対策ごとに図を使用

Sun Safety Action Steps

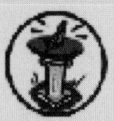
Limit Time in the Midday Sun
The sun's rays are strongest between 10 a.m. and 4 p.m. Whenever possible, limit exposure to the sun during these hours.

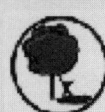
Seek Shade
Shade is a good source of protection, but keep in mind that shade structures (e.g., trees, umbrellas, canopies) do not offer complete sun protection. Remember the shadow rule: Watch Your Shadow. No Shadow, Seek Shade!

Wear a Hat
A hat with a wide brim offers good sun protection to eyes, ears, face, and the back of your neck — areas particularly prone to overexposure to the sun.

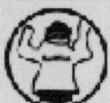
Cover Up
Wearing tightly woven, loose-fitting, and full-length clothing is a good way to protect your skin from the sun's UV rays.

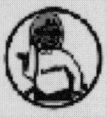
Wear Sunglasses that Block 99-100% of UV Radiation
Sunglasses that provide 99-100% UVA and UVB protection will greatly reduce sun exposure that can lead to cataracts and other eye damage. Check the label when buying sunglasses.

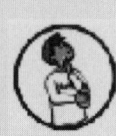
Always Use Sunscreen
Apply a broad spectrum sunscreen with a Sun Protection Factor (SPF) of at least 15 or higher liberally on exposed skin. Reapply every 2 hours, or after working, swimming, playing, or exercising outdoors. Even waterproof sunscreen can come off when you towel off, sweat, or spend extended periods of time in the water.

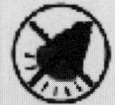
Avoid Sunlamps and Tanning Parlors
The light source from sunbeds and sunlamps damages the skin and unprotected eyes. It's a good idea to avoid artificial sources of UV light.

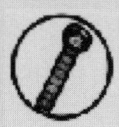
Watch for the UV Index
The UV Index provides important information to help you plan your outdoor activities in ways that prevent overexposure to the sun. Developed by the National Weather Service (NWS) and EPA, the UV Index is issued daily in selected cities across the United States.

http://www.epa.gov/sunwise/actionsteps.html

Glossary

brim	帽子のふち
broad spectrum sunscreen	広範囲の紫外線波長に有効な日焼け止め剤
canopy	天蓋，頭上を覆うもの
cataract	白内障
liberally	まんべんなく，十分に
prone to	～しがちな，～の傾向がある
tanning parlor	日焼けサロン
UV	紫外線 (ultraviolet), 380-200 nm の波長光 (UVA: 380-315 nm, UVB: 315-280 nm, UVC: 280 nm 以下)
UV Index	(http://www.epa.gov/sunwise/uvwhat.html) 紫外線指数

Expanding your vocabulary

Science texts often have words made up of affix parts. You should be able to guess the meaning of the word by considering the meaning of the parts.

sunglasses = sun + glasses → (1.   )
sunscreen = sun + screen → (2.   )
overexposure = over + exposure → (3.   )
sunlamps = sun + lamps → (4.   )
reapply = re + apply → (5.   )
unprotected = un + protected → (6.   )
waterproof = water + proof → (7.   )
outdoors = out + doors → (8.   )
midday = mid + day → (9.   )
sunbed = sun + bed → (10.   )

Reading the text for details (CD：トラック 14)

Listen to the CD reading of the text. After you have listened to it once, listen to it again but this time, try shadowing the reader. Practice this two or three times. Finally, do the following comprehension exercise. Decide whether the following statements are true (T) or false (F) or not stated (NS) in the text.

1. You should not spend too much time in the sun at midday.
2. A tree can completely protect you from exposure to ultraviolet rays.
3. Everyone should wear a hat.

4. UV exposure can cause damage to the eyes.
5. The EPA checks the type of protection offered by sunglasses.
6. The higher the SPF, the more protection the sunscreen can offer.
7. Unlike the sun, artificial UV light is safe.
8. The UV Index is a plan to help you enjoy outdoor life.

Check!

・SPF とは Sun Protection Factor の略号で Sun は太陽，Protection は防止，Factor は指数を意味し，紫外線による皮膚の炎症をどの程度防止できるかという目安の数値です．＊現在は SPF の最高値は 50+ です．

unlike 〜　〜とは違って

the more 〜, the more　〜すればするほどますます〜　　The more you practice, the more confident you will become. 練習すればするほど，自信も出てきますよ．

in ways that 〜，〜の（ような）やり方で　　in ways that prevent overexposure to the sun = in ways that you can prevent overexposure to the sun

Practicing a text feature : Imperative sentences

文中の表現を用いて，次の命令文を完成させなさい．

● Use English (1.　　) (2.　　).　できるだけ英語を使いなさい．

● Please (3.　　) (4.　　) (5.　　) that our weekly meeting has been rescheduled to 3:00 p.m. of November 2.　ウィークリーミーティングが 11 月 2 日の午後 3 時に変更されたことをお忘れなく．

● (6.　　) antiviral vendor's website for updates.　アップデートするにあたって，アンチウイルス・ベンダのウェブサイトをチェックしてください．

● (7.　　) touching these areas.　（図に示す）部分には触れないでください．＊マニュアルなどに頻出

● (8.　　) (9.　　) signs of asthma in children.　子供たちのぜんそくの兆候を注意して見ていてください．

● (10.　　) this cream each morning and night.　このクリームは，毎朝毎晩お使いください．＊薬などの使用法の指示

Try!

Make imperative sentences of your own to instruct someone about how to do something.

Saying it yourself （CD：トラック1）

Numbers are very important. Practice reading these sentences paying special attention to saying the numbers very clearly.

1. The sun's rays are strongest between 10 a.m. and 4 p.m.
2. Sunglasses that provide 99-100% UVA and UVB protection will greatly reduce sun exposure.
3. Apply a broad spectrum sunscreen with a Sun Protection Factor (SPF) of at least 15 or higher.
4. Reapply every 2 hours, or after working, swimming, playing, or exercising outdoors.

Try!

Make a sentence of your own including a number and practice reading it clearly.

英語あれこれノート

How you read an acronym depends on whether or not it can be pronounced as a word. How would you read the following? What do they stand for?

1. **UVA**
2. **UVB**
3. **EPA**
4. **NWS**
5. **SPF** （答えは巻末に）

Here are some others that can be read as words. Try reading them out loud.

JAMA	Journal of the American Medical Association
ASEAN	Association of Southeast Asian Nations
TEPCO	Tokyo Electric Power Company
MEXT	Ministry of Education, Culture, Sports, Science and Technology

Try!

Find an English acronym and what it represents.

Unit 1

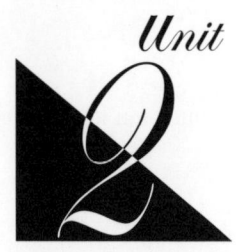

Genre: **Advice column**
Source: **The Times**

The Times

　イギリス（ロンドン）最大手の新聞社により 1785 年に創刊された The Times/The Sunday Times は，世界で最も有名な日刊紙のひとつである．日々の英国内におけるニュースをはじめ，国際ニュース，政治・議会関係，芸能・スポーツ，ビジネス関係，科学などの記事や論説が掲載されている．この新聞は長期にわたり，「冷静で，格調高く，洗練された，公正な，記事や論説を読者に提供している」という評価を得ており，現在では世界中の信頼を受けるイギリスの高級新聞紙となっている．オンライン版 Times/Sunday Times（London）（http://www.timesonline.co.uk/global/）は，誰でも無料で利用することができる．

Health Briefings

　The Times/The Sunday Times の健康欄には，健康に関するニュース，アドバイス，解説，食事や運動などに関する記事が掲載されている．この章では，健康に関する読者の疑問に医学の専門家が答える（解説する，説明する）Health Briefings をとりあげる．これは，読者が健康に関する疑問（症状やその継続期間，年齢，性別など）をメールで送る（http://www.timesonline.co.uk/section/0,,643,00.html）と，Dr Thomas Stuttaford が，個々のケースに対する回答ではなく一般的な疑問として回答（解説，説明）するというものである．この章では，2006 年 4 月 13 日オンライン版に掲載されたものをとりあげた．

Observing the text as a whole

　Look at the following page and think about its PAIL characteristics.　（**PAIL: P** = Purpose 文章の目的，**A** = Audience 文章の対象者，**I** = Information 情報の内容，**L** = Language features 文章の構成形態）

Genre:　　　　　　　Advice from an expert　専門家の助言
Purpose:　　　　　　To provide advice about health issues and questions　健康問題に関する専門家の助言を提供
Audience:　　　　　General public　一般の人々
Information:　　　　How to take advice　助言の取り入れ方
Language features: Paragraphs　段落構成
　　　　　　　　　　　Rather informal language (use of contractions such as "doesn't")　ややくだけた表現　（例：does not を doesn't にするなど）

＊ 11 ページ＜備考＞も参照すること．

The Times   April 13, 2006

Red wine good, red wine bad: which advice should I believe?

DR THOMAS STUTTAFORD

[Paragraph 1] A reader has heard that coffee is bad for health, so cut it from his diet. He exercises for an hour a day and, having read times2 on Monday, will avoid having sex on aircraft. He is left with one pleasure: red wine. But reports about its efficacy conflict. Who should he believe?

[Paragraph 2] Our reader's one hour of exercise a day is likely to improve his life expectancy, especially as it is brisk, but not violent. If it involves jogging, it should be done on grass rather than on the streets.

[Paragraph 3] The reader doesn't tell us his age, but in general it is better to avoid exercise in extreme temperatures. If it is very hot and muggy, or cold with a biting northeasterly blowing, reading the newspapers would serve his health better.

[Paragraph 4] He should also avoid exercise if he has flu, a severe cold or a temperature. Exercising when feverish occasionally precipitates apparently inexplicable sudden death in young people, often on the football field.

[Paragraph 5] The benefits of giving up coffee are not clear-cut. However, two cups a day wouldn't damage our reader's cardiovascular system, and might even improve it — it all depends on his genes. And if carefully timed it would not have kept him awake. The almost universally accepted belief is that modest amounts of alcoholic drink — and especially red wine — help to reduce deaths from ischaemic heart disease (coronary heart attacks). Alcohol in moderation can also be shown to increase longevity even after the benefits derived from the effect of alcohol on blood clotting and arterial disease have been removed from the equation. Unfortunately, if the alcohol intake rises above certain limits, the effect varies according to age, gender, race, family and lifestyle habits. In this instance the big advantages of alcohol to the cardiovascular system and the lesser ones to other organs are at first nullified, and later reversed.

[Paragraph 6] Alcohol, and especially red wine, increases the proportion of HDL (the good cholesterol) to LDL (the bad cholesterol). There is an overall decrease in the amount of pernicious LDL in modest drinkers. Alcohol also alters the clotting mechanism by decreasing platelet stickiness, and has a useful effect on the amount of fibrogen and fibrinolysis in the arteries.

[Paragraph 7] Over the past 30 years people have periodically suggested that the

scientific data and epidemiological studies that demonstrate the apparent advantages of modest drinking, as opposed to being a teetotaller, are illusory. The antis' hypothesis is that modest drinkers don't live longer because of the red wine or the occasional whisky or glass of beer. Their theory is that the apparent benefit of modest alcohol drinking conveyed by the drinker's improved survival times is related to characteristics in the lifestyle of teetotallers other than their rejection of alcohol.

[Paragraph 8] Among the factors that might undermine the health of teetotallers, other than a reluctance to drink, are a higher incidence of insomnia, anxious temperament, a greater tendency to be workaholics and to feel undervalued.

[Paragraph 9] The good news is that careful studies of the statistics of longevity are still encouraging to the modest drinker even after all these factors have been taken into account. These usually show that, as most of us hoped, a drink or two a day improves life expectation. Liver disease is a worry. Fortunately, only one liver in five is vulnerable and this vulnerability is especially apparent in young livers. If men were more careful than they are now to drink in the strictest moderation until they were over 35, and women until they were past the menopause, the statistics would look even better.

http://www.timesonline.co.uk/article/0,,8124-2131060,00.html

Glossary

antis	(antiの複数形) 学説，主義などに反対する人々
arterial	動脈の　　arterial disease　動脈関連疾患
clot	凝固する，(血等の) 塊　　blood clotting　血液凝固
fibrinolysis	線維素溶解
fibrogen	(血液中の) 線維素 (血栓の原因物質の1つ)
HDL (high density lipoprotein)	高比重リポ蛋白
ischaemic	虚血性の　　ischaemic heart disease　虚血性心疾患
LDL (low density lipoprotein)	低比重リポ蛋白
menopause	更年期，月経閉止 (期)
muggy	蒸し暑い
northeasterly	北東，北東の，北東に (ある)，北東へ (の)，北東から
nullify	無効にする
pernicious	有害な，破滅的な
stickiness	粘性
teetotaller	禁酒主義者
times2	イギリスで発行されている新聞 The Times と The Sunday Times のベスト記事のオンライン配信サイト
workaholic	仕事中毒の (人)

Expanding your vocabulary

Complete each sentence with the correct form of the most suitable word from the list. 次のリストから適切な単語を選び，正しい形にして文章を完成させなさい．

| arteries | clotting | feverish | insomnia | longevity |
| cardiovascular | epidemiological | inexplicable | ischaemia | moderation |

1. Some researchers claim that coffee is not good for the *heart and circulatory* system.
2. *Coagulating* of the blood can cause serious damage to the brain.
3. The causes of some diseases can be *difficult to explain*.
4. A healthy lifestyle can contribute to *living a long life*.
5. *Not eating or drinking too much* can help maintain optimal body weight.
6. A disease affecting the *vessels that carrying blood from the heart to the other parts of the body* can be life threatening.
7. *Transmission and control of disease* is important when a new disease is discovered.
8. The crying child seemed *to have a temperature*.
9. In hot summer, many people complain of *not being able to sleep*.
10. *Restriction of the blood supply* of the heart muscle causes angina pectoris.

Reading the text for details (CD：トラック 15)

Listen to the CD reading of the text. After you have listened to it once, listen to it again but this time, try shadowing the reader. Practice this two or three times. Finally, do the following comprehension exercise.

Identify the type of information being presented in each paragraph. 各パラグラフの内容を下から選びなさい．

Paragraph 1 :   *Paragraph 4* :   *Paragraph 7* :
Paragraph 2 :   *Paragraph 5* :   *Paragraph 8* :
Paragraph 3 :   *Paragraph 6* :   *Paragraph 9* :

A. Response to other items (drinking beverages) mentioned by reader
B. Mention of factors, such as age, related to exercising
C. Discussion of research related to benefits of alcohol consumption

D. Description of positive factors related to alcohol consumption
E. Question posed by a reader
F. Explanation of effects of alcohol
G. Continuing explanation of exercising and what should be avoided
H. Possible features of teetotallers' lifestyles
I. Response to one of the items (exercising) mentioned by reader

Practicing a text feature

Let's try summarizing and paraphrasing the text. Summarizing means saying the same thing but more concisely. Paraphrasing means expressing the same meaning using different words. When you want to use what someone else has written you should not copy the person's words. You should try to express what the person was trying to say using different words.

Complete the one-sentence summaries of the selected paragraphs. 文章を完成させて，下のそれぞれのパラグラフを一文で要約しましょう．

Paragraph 6 Alcohol can (*1.*   ) the ratio of (*2.*   ) to (*3.*   ) and help (*4.*   ) clotting in the arteries.

Paragraph 7 Some think that people who (*5.*   ) moderately live (*6.*   ) than teetotallers because of their (*7.*   ) rather than their (*8.*   ) drinking of alcohol.

Paragraph 8 Some (*9.*   ) features of (*10.*   ), such as not being able to sleep and feeling anxious, are not (*11.*   ) for the (*12.*   ).

Paragraph 9 However, while (*13.*   ) disease is a concern, modest (*14.*   ) for men until they are 35 and for women until menopause may be beneficial to (*15.*   ).

Saying it yourself   (CD：トラック 2)

Listen to the CD and fill in the blanks. Practice reading the passage aloud.

Alcohol, and especially red wine, (*1.*   ) the proportion of HDL (the good (*2.*   )) to LDL (the bad cholesterol). There is (*3.*   ) overall decrease in the amount (*4.*   ) pernicious LDL in modest drinkers. Alcohol (*5.*   ) alters the clotting mechanism by (*6.*   ) platelet stickiness, and has a useful (*7.*   ) on the amount of fibrogen and fibrinolysis (*8.*   ) the arteries.

英語あれこれノート

One of the effective ways to expand your vocabulary is to learn words and phrases in their context of use. Sometimes these contexts extend over an entire sentence. In such a case, it would be more efficient to learn the framework of the sentence. Check how the following frameworks are used in the original text and then try using them to make sentences of your own.

even after ～ have been removed from the equation: ～を計算式から除外したとしても

the advantages of ～ are nullified: ～の効果は（逆の効果を誘発する要因と相殺されて）無効になる

even after all these factors have been taken into account: これらの要因を考慮に入れたとしても

<備考>

健康に関する情報のとらえかた

　我々はメディアを通して日常的に健康に関する情報にさらされています．この記事では，アルコールの有効性についても述べられており，一般の読者は，この記事を読んで，自分のアルコール摂取を正当化するために利用するかもしれません．では，医療従事者になろうとする薬学生は，この内容をどうとらえるべきでしょうか．科学者・専門家として，その情報を鵜呑みにすることなく，自分の知識と照らし合わせ，内容の是非を判断する姿勢をもつ必要があります．

　医療の担い手になろうとする皆さんが，この記事の読者であったなら，「確かに有効性も報告されているが，本当に身体に良いと言えるのか？」「どのような成分が，どのような機序で，その効果を発揮するのだろう？」「適量はどのくらいか？」「有害性はないのか？」などの疑問を抱きながら読み，さらに，その科学的根拠を調べてみてください．

英語の記事によく見られる表現

　今回の記事の中には性に関する表現がジョークとして使用されています．日本とは異なり，海外ではこの手のジョークを軽く笑って受け流すという文化的背景を理解する一助となるよう，原文をそのまま掲載しています．

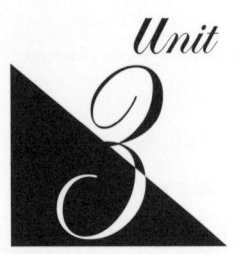

Genre: **Public health notification**
Source: **Food and Drug Administration**

FDA（Food and Drug Administration） 米国食品医薬品局

　米国厚生省に属する公衆保健のための行政機関で，食品や医薬品をはじめ，医療器具，化粧品，放射線を発する製品，動物用の餌や医薬品などの安全に関する責任を負っている．FDA は，ホームページ（http://www.fda.gov/）で，監視下の製品が正しく使用されるための情報を提供している．この章でとりあげる公衆衛生通知（public health notification）は，医療器具を安全に取り扱うための情報として発信されているものである．

　FDA はこの通知の科学的エビデンスとして，感染症対策総合研究所である米国疾病予防管理センター CDC（Centers for Disease Control and Prevention）が公開している MMWR（Morbidity and Mortality Weekly Report，週間疾病率死亡率報告）Dispatch を引用している．MMWR Dispatch は，毎週米国の監視対象とされている感染症の発生状況を分析した報告書である．CDC は，各州の公衆衛生局から報告された情報をもとに，最新の研究成果などと合わせて，翌週に web（http://www.cdc.gov/mmwr/）上に公表している．

Observing the text as a whole

Look at the following page and think about its PAIL characteristics. （**PAIL**: P = Purpose　文章の目的，**A** = Audience　文章の対象者，**I** = Information　情報の内容，**L** = Language features　文章の構成形態）

Genre: Official warning or notice on public health issue　公衆衛生に関する公式の警告および通知

Purpose: To warn people about some health-related issue　健康に関して警告する

Audience: Healthcare practitioners　医療関係者
Those in the general public affected by the issue　この問題の影響を受ける一般の人々

Information: Description of problem and instructions about what to do　問題の説明と対処に関する指示

Language features: Open letter to healthcare practitioners　医療関係者への公開書簡
Formal language　フォーマルな表現

FDA Public Health Notification: Fungal Keratitis Infections Related to Contact Lens Use

Updated: May 31, 2006

Original Publication date: April 10, 2006

Dear Healthcare Practitioner:

We are updating the Preliminary Public Health Notification of April 10, 2006, with new information on the recent increase in reports of a rare but serious fungal infection of the eye in soft contact lens wearers in the U.S. The infection, a fungal keratitis caused by the *Fusarium* fungus, may cause vision loss requiring corneal transplants.

New Information

On May 15, 2006, **Bausch and Lomb announced its decision to permanently remove all ReNu with MoistureLoc products worldwide. As previously recommended, consumers should stop using ReNu with MoistureLoc immediately.**

On May 19, 2006, the CDC released an MMWR Dispatch updating its on-going multistate investigation into *Fusarium* keratitis occurring in contact lens wearers. This update can be found at http://www.cdc.gov/mmwr/preview/mmwrhtml/mm55d519a1.htm. The CDC findings continue to show an increased risk for *Fusarium* keratitis linked to using Bausch and Lomb's ReNu with MoistureLoc in the month prior to the onset of infection.

Both the Food and Drug Administration (FDA) and the Centers for Disease Control and Prevention (CDC) continue to investigate reports of fungal keratitis in an effort to determine all contributing factors and/or products that place contact lens wearers at increased risk for *Fusarium* keratitis.

At this time, we do not expect our recommendations to change since Bausch and Lomb has permanently removed all ReNu with MoistureLoc worldwide. However, if we identify additional risk factors, or if we have new recommendations for the clinical community or contact lens wearers, we will provide an update.

Recommendations

For healthcare providers:

- Advise patients to stop using Bausch and Lomb ReNu with MoistureLoc products immediately, discard all remaining MoistureLoc solution and use an alternative cleaning/disinfecting product.
- If a patient presents with a microbial keratitis, consider that a fungal infection may be involved.
- Prior to initiating immediate treatment, an eye care professional should obtain a specimen for laboratory analysis.
- Report cases of fungal keratitis in contact lens wearers to FDA as noted below.

For contact lens wearers:

- Stop using Bausch and Lomb ReNu with MoistureLoc products and discard all remaining MoistureLoc solution including partially used or unopened bottles.
- Consult your eye care professional concerning use of an appropriate alternative cleaning/disinfecting product.
- Consider performing a "rub and rinse" lens cleaning method, rather than a no rub method, regardless of which cleaning/disinfecting solution used, in order to minimize the number of germs and reduce the chances of infection.
- Continue to follow proper lens care practices:
  - Wash hands with soap and water, and dry (lint-free method) before handling lenses.
  - Wear and replace lenses according to the schedule prescribed by the doctor.
  - Follow the specific lens cleaning and storage guidelines from the doctor and the solution manufacturer.
  - Keep the contact lens case clean and replace every 3-6 months.
  - Remove the lenses and consult your doctor immediately if you experience symptoms such as redness, pain, tearing, increased light sensitivity, blurry vision, discharge or swelling.

FDA Advice to Patients on this topic can be found at http://www.fda.gov/cdrh/medicaldevicesafety/atp/041006-keratitis.html.

Background

In an MMWR Dispatch dated April 10, 2006, CDC stated that it received reports of 109 cases of suspected fungal keratitis in 17 different states. Although the majority of case patients have yet to be interviewed, complete data are available for 30 of them. Twenty-eight of the 30 wore soft contact lenses. Preliminary information obtained by CDC from patient interviews indicates that 26 of these patients remembered which products they used, and that all 26 reported using a Bausch & Lomb ReNu brand contact lens solution in the month prior to the onset of infection. Patients reported using a variety of different ReNu types from multiple different product lots. Five of the patients reported using other solutions in addition to the ReNu product. Nine of the patients reported wearing lenses overnight, a known risk factor for microbial keratitis. Eight required corneal transplantation. Strain typing of the organism is ongoing. This document can be found at http://www.cdc.gov/mmwr/preview/mmwrhtml/mm55d410a1.htm.

CDC and FDA are investigating these case reports. Also, investigations by CDC, state and local health departments, FDA, and manufacturers of contact lens solutions are underway to define specific behaviors or products that place contact lens wearers at increased risk for *Fusarium* keratitis.

Clusters of *Fusarium* keratitis were reported among contact lens users in Asia beginning in February 2006. At that time, Bausch & Lomb voluntarily suspended sales of its ReNu multipurpose solutions in Singapore and Hong Kong, pending their investigations, after multiple reports of *Fusarium* keratitis among contact lens users there.

http://www.fda.gov/cdrh/safety/041006-keratitis.html

Glossary

biometrics	バイオメトリクス，生体認証（顔，指紋，目の虹彩などで個人を見分ける技術）
blurry	（目が）かすむ
cornea	角膜（黒目の上を覆う透明な膜）
corticosteroid	副腎皮質ステロイド
disinfect	消毒する，殺菌する
immunocompromised	免疫無防備状態の（免疫システムが損なわれた状態）
immunodeficiency	免疫不全（症）
initiate	開始する
keratitis	角膜炎（角膜に細菌やウイルスなどが感染して炎症がおきた状態）
lint	糸くず，ほこり
medication	投薬
multipurpose	多目的の
notification	公告，公告文，告示
ocular	眼球の，視覚の
prescribe	処方する
redness	発赤

regimen	療法，投与計画，措置
require	～を必要とする
rinse	ゆすぐ
systemic	全身の
transplantation	移植

Expanding your vocabulary

Many adjectives have "-al" as an ending. This rule of thumb applies even to technical terms. How are these words used in the following sentences?

| additional | clinical | corneal | medical | partial | radiological |
| annual | conjunctival | fungal | microbial | professional | topical |

1. Athlete's foot is a (　　) infection that usually affects the toes.
2. (　　) organizations, such as the Japan Medical Society and Japan Pharmaceutical Association, aim at the advancement and development of those working in their fields.
3. He needed a (　　) transplant due to the damage from the keratitis.
4. Various (　　) technologies, such as ultrasound and computed tomography, can be used to detect and diagnose disease.
5. (　　) research is needed to check whether the solution actually caused the infection.
6. Due to only (　　) recovery from the injury, he had to continue the rehabilitation.
7. The (　　) incidence of the disease has increased as the population of users increased.
8. The pharmacist recommended a (　　) ointment to stop the itching.
9. (　　) trials are used to test new medical devices or medicines before they are approved for general use.
10. The redness of her eyes was due to an infection of the (　　) membrane.
11. (　　) infections are caused by microorganisms such as Escherichia coli.
12. They developed a new (　　) device to help improve hearing.

Reading the text for details   (CD：トラック 16)

Listen to the CD reading of the text. After you have listened to it once, listen to it again but this time, try shadowing the reader. Practice this two or three times. Finally, do the following comprehension exercise.

Decide on whether the following information is true (T) or false (F) or not stated (NS) in the text. Give the section to which you referred to make your decision. 次の内容が本文と一致するかどうか判断し（T: true ＝ 本文の内容と合致する，F: false ＝ 本文の内容と合致しない，NS: not stated ＝ 本文に書かれていない），判断材料となったセクション（Opening address (Dear Healthcare Practitioner:)，New Information，Recommendations）を答えなさい．

1. The fungal infection described in this public health notification is a very common problem with people who use contact lens.
2. The company decided to stop selling the product that caused the fungal infection.
3. The CDC has also been conducting investigations on all contact wearers.
4. The FDA decided to ban the use of the product causing the problem.
5. If a case of fungal keratitis is found by a healthcare professional, it should be reported to the CDC.
6. A professional should start treatment as soon as possible and conduct laboratory analysis later.
7. Japanese contact lens wearers should stop using the problem products.
8. Contact lenses should be worn and replaced as instructed by the doctor.
9. A new contact lens case should be obtained after three to six months.
10. Symptoms that require professional help include increased sensitivity to light and difficulty seeing due to blurriness.

Practicing a text feature

FDA, CDC, Bausch and Lomb のおのおのは，起こった問題に対してどのように行動したでしょうか．このように情報が錯綜しているときは，おのおのが主語になっている文を探すことで，アウトラインが見えてきます．

1. FDA, CDC, FDA and CDC, Bausch and Lomb が主語になっている文を探し，異なる4色のマーカーでハイライトをつけてみましょう．（注：本文中に出てくる We に注意！ We は，上の4者のうちどれを指しますか？）

2. ハイライトをつけた文をヒントにして，次のような 5W1H（誰が，いつ，どこで，何のために，何を，どのように，どうした）の表をノートに完成させなさい．

Who 誰が	When いつ	Where どこで	What 何をした・する	Why 何のために	How どのように
FDA	A.	B.	C.		D.
	E.		F.		
CDC	G.		H.		
	I.	J.	K.		
FDA and CDC	L.		M.	N.	
	O.		P.		
Bausch and Lomb	Q.	R.	S.		
	T.	U.	V.		W.

3. 時間の経過をたどってみましょう．どのような順で事態が推移したか確認してみましょう．

4. それぞれのアクションがとられたのは何のためか（Why）考えてみましょう．

Saying it yourself （CD：トラック3）

Listen to the CD and practice reading the following passage aloud. Note in particular how to read the postal address, phone number, e-mail address and URL.

If you have questions about this notification, please contact Nancy Pressly, Office of Surveillance and Biometrics (HFZ-510), 1350 Piccard Drive, Rockville, Maryland, 20850, Fax at 301-594-2968, or by e-mail at phann@cdrh.fda.gov. You may also leave a voice mail message at 301-594-0650 and we will return your call as soon as possible.

FDA medical device Public Health Notifications are available on the Internet at http://www.fda.gov/cdrh/safety.html.

英語あれこれノート

This text reports that "microbial keratitis" can be a serious problem with contact lens users. The word "keratitis" means "inflammation of the cornea." The "itis" ending, which means "inflammation," appears in many terms related to diseases. Here are some other types of diseases. Match them with their meaning in Japanese.

-itis は，炎症を表す接尾辞です．次の英語で記された病名を日本語と結び付けてみましょう． （答えは巻末に）

1. appendicitis
2. arthritis
3. conjunctivitis
4. dermatitis
5. gastritis
6. hepatitis
7. encephalitis
8. stomatitis
9. nephritis
10. cystitis

a. 胃炎
b. 肝炎
c. 関節炎
d. 結膜炎
e. 口内炎
f. 腎炎
g. 虫垂炎
h. 脳炎
i. 皮膚炎
j. 膀胱炎

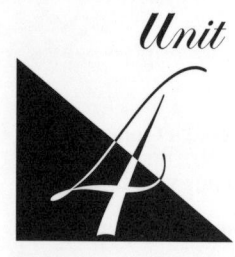

Genre: **Wiki**
Source: **Wikipedia**

Wikipedia

ウィキペディア（Wikipedia）は，ウィキ + encyclopedia（百科事典），すなわち，米国フロリダ州にある非営利団体ウィキメディア財団によりインターネット上で作成・公開されているオープンコンテント方式の多言語百科事典である（http://ja.wikipedia.org/）. 2001年1月に英語のみで始められたこのプロジェクトは，現在，150 を超える言語で 3,300,000 項目以上に達する巨大辞典となっている．基本方針に賛同するならば，だれでも記事を投稿したり編集したりすることができる．更新されたページは，編集者により査読・監視されてはいるものの，その膨大さゆえにすべてに対応でき得ているかが問題視されているのも現状である．利用者は，記事によってはその内容を鵜呑みにするのではなく，それが正しい情報であるか否かを判断する能力が要求されるかもしれない．

Observing the text as a whole

Look at the following page and think about its PAIL characteristics. （**PAIL**: **P** = Purpose 文章の目的，**A** = Audience 文章の対象者，**I** = Information 情報の内容，**L** = Language features 文章の構成形態）

Genre:	Encyclopedic information 百科事典
Purpose:	To describe a phenomenon 言葉の意味の説明
Audience:	General public 一般の人々
Information:	Explanation of headache, its pathophysiology and treatment 頭痛の説明，病気の成因と治療法
Language features:	Paragraphs 段落構成
	Rather informal language ややくだけた表現 （use of contractions such as "doesn't"）

Headache

From Wikipedia, the free encyclopedia

A headache (medically known as cephalalgia, sometimes spelled as cephalgia) is a condition of pain in the head; sometimes neck or upper back pain may also be interpreted as a headache. It ranks amongst the most common local pain complaints.

Headaches have a wide variety of causes, ranging from eye strain, sinusitis and tension to life-threatening conditions such as encephalitis, meningitis, cerebral aneurysms and brain tumors. When the headache occurs in conjunction with a head injury the cause is usually quite evident; however, many causes are more unclear. The most common type of headache is a tension headache. Some experience headaches when dehydrated; caffeine withdrawal is another common cause.

Treatment of uncomplicated headache is usually symptomatic with over-the-counter painkillers such as aspirin, paracetamol (acetaminophen) or ibuprofen, although some specific forms of headaches (e.g. migraine) may demand other, more suitable treatment.

Pathophysiology

The brain itself is not sensitive to pain, because it lacks pain-sensitive nerve fibers. Several areas of the head can hurt, including a network of nerves which extends over the scalp and certain nerves in the face, mouth, and throat. The meninges and the blood vessels do have pain perception. Headache often results from traction to or irritation of the meninges and blood vessels. The muscles of the head may similarly be sensitive to pain.

Treatment

Not all headaches require medical attention, and respond with simple analgesics (painkillers) such as paracetamol/acetaminophen or members of the NSAID class (such as aspirin/acetylsalicylic acid or ibuprofen).

In recurrent unexplained headaches, healthcare professionals may recommend keeping a "headache diary" with entries on type of headache, associated symptoms, precipitating and aggravating factors. This may reveal specific patterns, such as an association with medication, menstruation and absenteeism.

Some forms of headache may be amenable to preventative treatment, such as migraine. On the whole, long-term use of painkillers is discouraged as this may lead to "rebound headaches" on withdrawal. Caffeine, a vasoconstrictor, is sometimes prescribed or recommended, as a remedy or supplement to pain killers in the case of extreme migraine. This has led to the development of Tylenol Ultra, a paracetamol/caffeine analgesic. One popular herbal treatment for migraines is Feverfew.

http://en.wikipedia.org/wiki/Headache

Wikipedia "Headache"

Glossary

absenteeism	常習的欠席，欠勤
acetaminophen	アセトアミノフェン（解熱鎮痛剤）
acetylsalicylic acid	アセチルサリチル酸，アスピリン（解熱鎮痛剤）
amenable	～に反応する
amongst	～の間で
analgesia	無痛覚症（痛覚欠如，強い侵害刺激を与えてもほとんど痛覚を感じない状態）
aneurysm	動脈瘤（動脈の壁が局所的にこぶ状に拡張した状態で，原因の多くは動脈硬化症や外傷などによる．次第に増大し破裂することがある）
caffeine withdrawal	カフェイン禁断（頭痛）（コーヒーなどカフェイン含有飲料を大量に常用している人の一部にみられる肉体依存様の禁断症状．偏頭痛様の症状が現われる）
cephalalgia/cephalgia/cephalea	頭痛（医学用語，headache と同じ）
encephalitis	脳炎（髄膜炎の症状に加え脳実質内に炎症が及んだ状態で，意識障害や片麻痺，半盲，失語といった脳の局所に障害が生じる）
eyestrain	眼精疲労
feverfew	夏白菊（ナツシロギク，欧米では鎮痛効果があるとして片頭痛に有効とされているハーブ）
healthcare	医療
herbal	薬草の
ibuprofen	イブプロフェン（解熱鎮痛剤）
meninges	髄膜（脳や脊髄を覆う薄い膜）（meninx の複数形）
meningitis	髄膜炎（髄膜の中を流れる脳脊髄液中に細菌，ウィルス，真菌類が進入する事により発症する，炎症が脳の表面だけで脳実質に及んでいない状態）
menstruation	月経，生理
NSAID（nonsteroidal anti-inflammatory drug）	非ステロイド系抗炎症薬（ステロイドではない鎮痛，解熱，抗炎症作用を有する薬剤の総称）
painkiller	鎮痛薬（pain reliever と同じ）
paracetamol	パラセタモール（解熱鎮痛剤）
precipitate	沈殿（物）
rebound	跳ね返り，反発
scalp	頭皮
sinusitis	副鼻腔炎（アレルギーや感染により副鼻腔に炎症がおきた状態．慢性の副鼻腔炎がいわゆる蓄膿症）
traction	けんいん性の
Tylenol ®	タイレノール（商品名，米国で市販されている解熱鎮痛剤）
vasoconstrictor	血管収縮薬

Expanding your vocabulary

次の 1 ～ 10 までの英単語を同じ意味を持つ日本語（a ～ h），および，英語の同義語（A ～ H）と結び付けなさい．

1. aggravating
2. preventative
3. symptomatic
4. uncomplicated
5. unexplained
6. analgesic
7. dehydrated
8. pathophysiology
9. migraine
10. cerebral

a. 病態生理学
b. 鎮痛剤
c. 脳の
d. 対症状の
e. 一層悪化させる
f. 単純な
g. 脱水状態になっている
h. 片頭痛
i. 予防する
j. 解明されていない

A. unclear
B. dry
C. headache
D. worsening
E. simple
F. narcotic
G. preventive
H. physiology of abnormal states
I. brain
J. concerned with symptoms

Reading the text for details

Match the beginning of the sentence with the best ending below, based on the information in the text. 本文を参照して，1〜8の主語に対応する述部をA〜Hから選びなさい．

1. Some specific headaches
2. NSAIDS
3. Preventative medication
4. The most common type of headache
5. The brain
6. Inflammation of the meninges or the brain
7. Long-term uses of analgesia
8. Headaches

A. may be an effective way of treating migraine.
B. result from a variety of causes.
C. are usually used for treatment of uncomplicated headaches.
D. exhibits little sensitivity to pain.
E. may cause rebound headaches on withdrawal.
F. may be a warning signal of more serious disorders.
G. is one of the common causes of headache.
H. is a tension headache.

Practicing a text feature

百科事典は，何か調べたい事柄があるときに，ごく大雑把な情報を提供してくれます．欲しい情報がどこにあるかをすばやく見つけるには，サブセクションを示すサブタイトルと各パラグラフのトピックセンテンス（パラグラフの最初のセンテンス）に注目します．

1. 次のことを知りたいときに，どのサブセクションを読みますか？
   a. 頭の痛みを感じるとき，体の中ではいったい何が起こっているのだろう？
   b. 頭痛の治療法にはどのようなものがあるのだろう？
   c. 頭痛とは，医学的にどのような現象を指し示すのだろう？

2. 次のことを調べたいときに，どのトピックセンテンスを読みますか？
   a. 頭痛の病態（どこで痛みを感じているのか？）
   b. 頭痛が起こる原因
   c. 頭痛の予防法
   d. 頭痛の医学的定義
   e. 頭痛の治療法

Try!

3. 2. の a-e の中で，特に興味のある項目をひとつ選び，セクション内容をまとめて発表しなさい．

Saying it yourself （CD：トラック4）

There are many disease and medicine names that are difficult to pronounce. Listen to the following passage carefully and practice reading it as smoothly and as quickly as possible.

Not all headaches require medical attention, and respond with simple analgesics (painkillers) such as paracetamol/acetaminophen or members of the NSAID class (such as aspirin/acetylsalicylic acid or ibuprofen).

Some forms of headache may be amenable to preventative treatment, such as migraine. On the whole, long-term use of painkillers is discouraged as this may lead to "rebound headaches" on withdrawal. Caffeine, a vasoconstrictor, is sometimes prescribed or recommended, as a remedy or supplement to pain killers in the case of extreme migraine. This has led to the development of Tylenol® Ultra, a paracetamol/caffeine analgesic. One popular herbal treatment for migraines is Feverfew.

英語あれこれノート

Many verbs are used in V-ing and V-ed forms as adjectives. Here are some examples from the text. 次の単語はいずれも，動詞に -ing または -ed がついて形容詞となったものです．

...that place contact lens wearers at **increased** risk for Fusarium *keratitis*.
...it received reports of 109 cases of **suspected** fungal keratitis...
...FDA will be sharting **reported** information with CDC...

形容詞	もとの動詞
aggravating　悪化させるような	aggravate　〜を（さらに）悪化させる
dehydrated　脱水状態（になっている）	dehydrate　脱水状態になる，乾燥する
uncomplicated (un + complicated)　複雑でない，単純な	complicate　複雑にする
unexplained (un + explained)　説明されていない，解明されていない	explain　説明する
recommended　推奨の	recommend　推奨する
threatening　脅かすような	threaten　脅かす

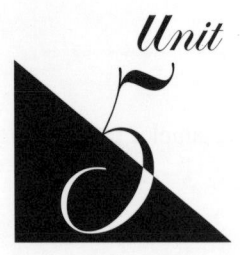

Genre: **Public announcement**
Source: **Tokyo Metropolitan Government**

東京都における廃棄物の状況および使用済み注射針回収事業

　日本全国の一般廃棄物の総排出量は，5000万トンを超える．その約1割は，東京都が占めるが，ごみに関する意識は非常に高いものがあり，その排出量は，過去10年着実に減少の道をたどっている．都民のごみに対する関心も高まりをみせ，各自治会による集団回収も活発に行われている．さらに独創的なのは，医療廃棄物の回収事業である．高齢化社会の進展に伴い，慢性疾患の増加や自宅での医療受診の要望に対応するため，これまで医療機関で行われてきた医療行為が，在宅においても実施されるようになり，従来，医療機関より排出されていた注射器等の医療廃棄物が，家庭からも多く排出されるようになった．そのため，ごみ収集時における針刺し事故の防止が課題となっており，平成14年11月，東京都からの働きかけを契機に，薬局による使用済み注射針の回収事業が杉並区・練馬区で開始した．現在，この事業は，都内23区および多摩地域で実施され，今後の更なる拡大が期待されている．

Observing the text as a whole

Look at the following page and think about its PAIL characteristics. （**PAIL: P** = Purpose　文章の目的，**A** = Audience　文章の対象者，**I** = Information　情報の内容，**L** = Language features　文章の構成形態）

Genre:	Public announcement　公告
Purpose:	To explain to the public what the local government is doing and what rules and regulations now apply　地方行政の政策実行内容および関連の規則，規定を説明
Audience:	General public　一般の人々
Information:	Description of waste and recycling by the Tokyo Metropolitan Government　東京都のゴミ対策，リサイクル運動の記述
Language features:	Paragraphs　段落構成
	Visual aids to present data and support explanations　データその他の提示に視覚資料を使用

Environment of Tokyo in 2005

Waste Categories

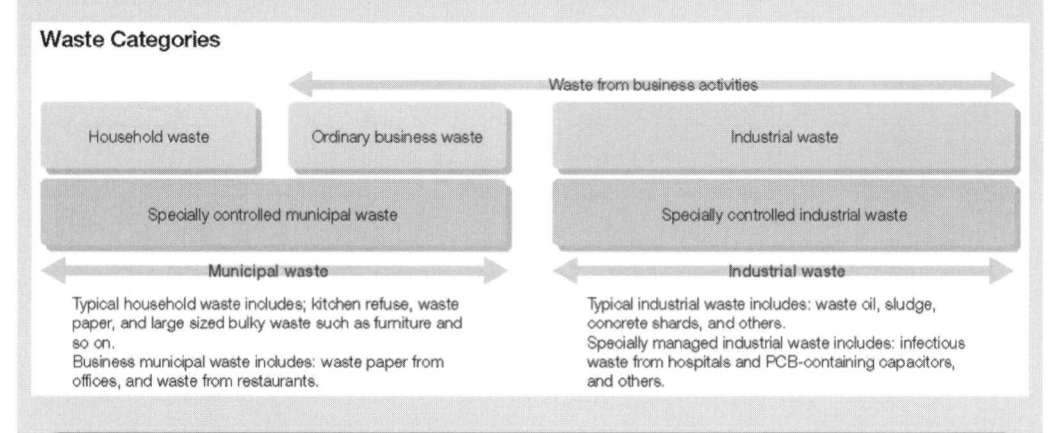

```
←———————————— Waste from business activities ————————————→
┌──────────────────┬──────────────────────┐  ┌──────────────────────────────────────┐
│ Household waste  │ Ordinary business    │  │ Industrial waste                     │
│                  │ waste                │  │                                      │
├──────────────────┴──────────────────────┤  ├──────────────────────────────────────┤
│ Specially controlled municipal waste    │  │ Specially controlled industrial waste│
└─────────────────────────────────────────┘  └──────────────────────────────────────┘
←———————— Municipal waste ————————→           ←———————— Industrial waste ————————→
```

Typical household waste includes; kitchen refuse, waste paper, and large sized bulky waste such as furniture and so on.
Business municipal waste includes: waste paper from offices, and waste from restaurants.

Typical industrial waste includes: waste oil, sludge, concrete shards, and others.
Specially managed industrial waste includes: infectious waste from hospitals and PCB-containing capacitors, and others.

Present State of Municipal Waste

The total municipal waste generated nationwide in 2002 amounted to 51.61 million tons.

Meanwhile, total waste (preliminary figures) generated in Tokyo Prefecture overall in FY2003 was roughly constant at 5.17 million tons.

Of this, waste generated in the 23 wards of Tokyo was 3.82 million tons, that generated in Tama region was 1.34 million tons, and that generated on the islands of Tokyo was 20,000 tons, all holding steady at previous levels.

Municipal waste is roughly divided into combustible waste, noncombustible waste and bulky waste as well as recyclable waste, which is converted directly to resources through sorted collection.

In addition, group collection by local resident associations and other organizations is also being carried out actively.

Volume of municipal waste by type in Tokyo (FY2003)

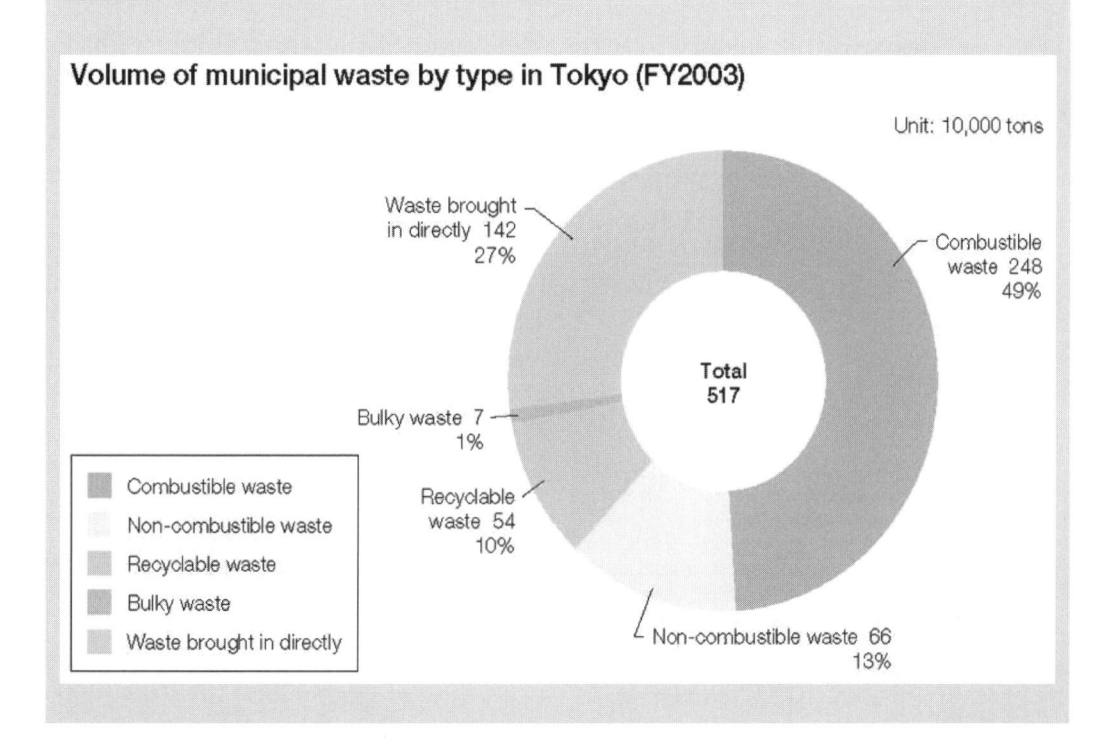

Unit: 10,000 tons

Total 517

- Combustible waste 248 — 49%
- Waste brought in directly 142 — 27%
- Non-combustible waste 66 — 13%
- Recyclable waste 54 — 10%
- Bulky waste 7 — 1%

Trends in waste volume in Tokyo (including recyclable waste)

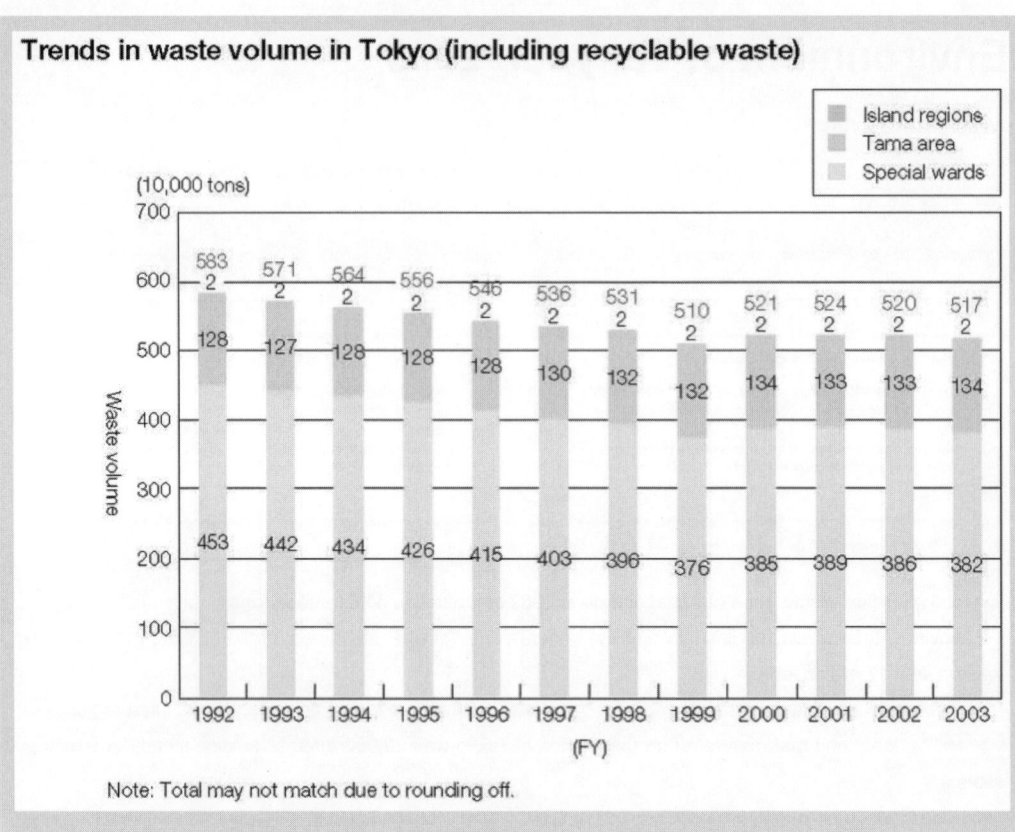

Legend: Island regions, Tama area, Special wards

(10,000 tons)

FY	Special wards	Tama area	Island regions	Total
1992	453	128	2	583
1993	442	127	2	571
1994	434	128	2	564
1995	426	128	2	556
1996	415	128	2	546
1997	403	130	2	536
1998	396	132	2	531
1999	376	132	2	510
2000	385	134	2	521
2001	389	133	2	524
2002	386	133	2	520
2003	382	134	2	517

Note: Total may not match due to rounding off.

Trends in final disposal volume of municipal waste in Tokyo

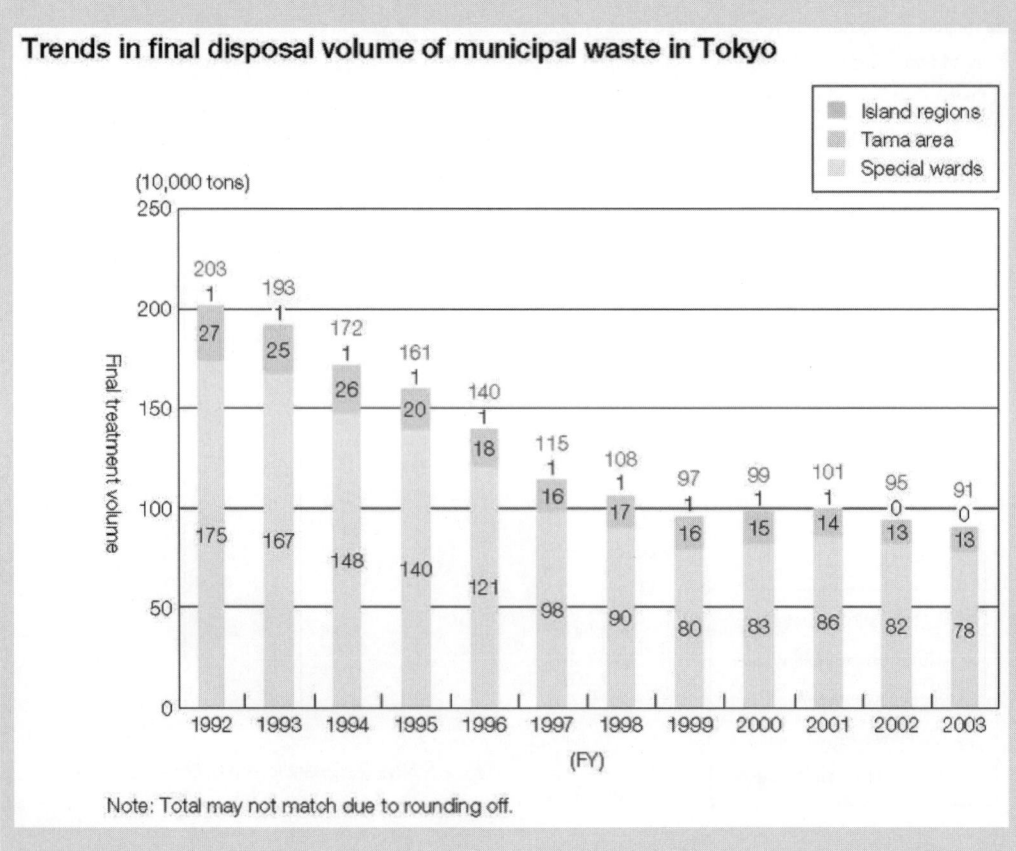

Legend: Island regions, Tama area, Special wards

(10,000 tons)

FY	Special wards	Tama area	Island regions	Total
1992	175	27	1	203
1993	167	25	1	193
1994	148	26	1	172
1995	140	20	1	161
1996	121	18	1	140
1997	98	16	1	115
1998	90	17	1	108
1999	80	16	1	97
2000	83	15	1	99
2001	86	14	1	101
2002	82	13	0	95
2003	78	13	0	91

Note: Total may not match due to rounding off.

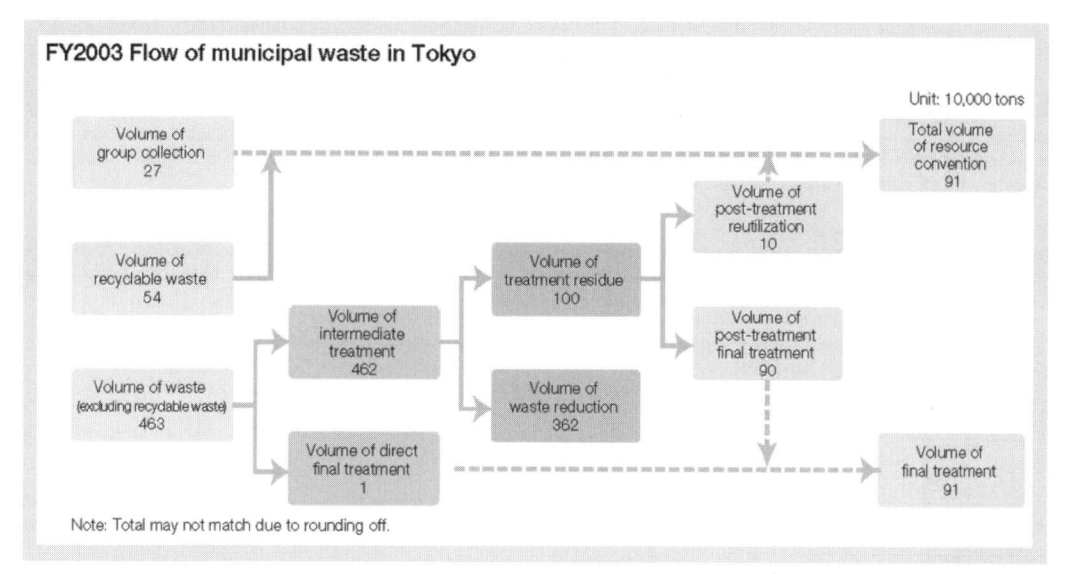

FY2003 Flow of municipal waste in Tokyo

Unit: 10,000 tons

- Volume of group collection: 27
- Volume of recyclable waste: 54
- Volume of waste (excluding recyclable waste): 463
- Volume of intermediate treatment: 462
- Volume of direct final treatment: 1
- Volume of treatment residue: 100
- Volume of waste reduction: 362
- Volume of post-treatment reutilization: 10
- Volume of post-treatment final treatment: 90
- Total volume of resource convention: 91
- Volume of final treatment: 91

Note: Total may not match due to rounding off.

注

Total volume of resource convention = Total volume of recycled waste
Volume of final treatment = Total volume of finally remained and dumped waste
Volume of waste reduction = Reduced waste volume by the intermediate waste processing

Reducing Waste Generation and Recycling

The Basic Law for Promotion of a Recycling-based Society was enacted in May 2000 to provide a basic framework for a comprehensive and strategic approach to waste and recycling issues. To build a recycling society promoting waste control and recycling, the roles of citizens, business enterprises and administrative authorities must be clearly defined, and their activities and coordination of efforts reinforced.

The citizen must fulfill his or her responsibility as a waste producer and take appropriate action in everyday life, such as selection of products that minimize waste production from the purchase stage. Founded on the policy of extended producer responsibility, business enterprises must promote systems and mechanisms that reduce waste. TMG must work aggressively to organize a new recycling system, build wide-area mechanisms and support municipal government efforts.

Promotion of self-collection by business enterprises

Self-collection by business enterprises is defined as the collection of products, containers, etc., produced and marketed by the manufacturers and vendors themselves and is one of the practical applications of extended producer responsibility (EPR). This is expected to boost environment-awareness and reduction of waste from the level of production design and manufacturing, such as the development of products that are easy to recycle or products that produce little waste.

At present, this is required for products such as air conditioners, television sets, refrigerators and washing machines under the Specified Household Appliance Recycling Law and personal computers and compact rechargeable batteries, that are designated as products to be recycled under the Law for Promotion of Effective Utilization of Resources.

TMG has conducted a review of new mechanisms for self-collection by manufacturers and has encouraged the national government to revise the law.

In FY2004, we carried out a proposal request to the government for radical revisions in Containers and Packaging Recycling Law and aid for the collection business of home medical care waste (used syringes) by the Tokyo Pharmaceutical Association.

Collection of Syringes by Pharmacies

Close-up ENVIRONMENTAL STRATEGY

Collection of used syringes by pharmacies began in November 2002 under the initiative of the Tokyo Pharmaceutical Association, under the auspices of TMG. Starting in Suginami and Nerima wards, it has expanded since 2003 and a total of 20 wards, 10 cities, and 3 towns carry out the collection of syringes as of the end of FY2004.

Municipalities covered (at the end of FY2004)
Chuo, Minato, Shinjuku, Bunkyo, Taito, Sumida, Koto, Shinagawa, Meguro, Setagaya, Shibuya, Nakano, Suginami, Toshima, Kita, Itabashi, Nerima, Adachi, Katsushika, and Edogawa wards, Hachioji, Musashino, Ome, Kodaira, Higashimurayama, Fussa, Komae, Higashikurume, Hamura, and Akiruno cities, and Mizuho, Hinode, and Okutama towns.

Collected items
Syringes purchased at pharmacies by patients treated at home and disposed of as in-home hospital waste.
Program organizers
Tokyo Pharmaceutical Association and local chapters of the Association
Program profile
Syringes purchased by in-home patients at pharmacies and disposed of after use are collected by pharmacies for appropriate processing.
Outline of the collection operation
1. When patients purchase syringes at pharmacies, containers for placing used syringes are distributed to purchasers.
2. After use, the patient brings the container containing used syringes to the pharmacy where they were purchased.
3. The representatives of pharmacies bring the collected containers to the regional control centers that store drugs and other pharmaceutical products when they come to pick up necessary drugs and products.
4. Containers brought in by pharmacy representatives are stored at the center and handed over to operators licensed for processing special-control industrial wastes for collection, transport and correct disposal.

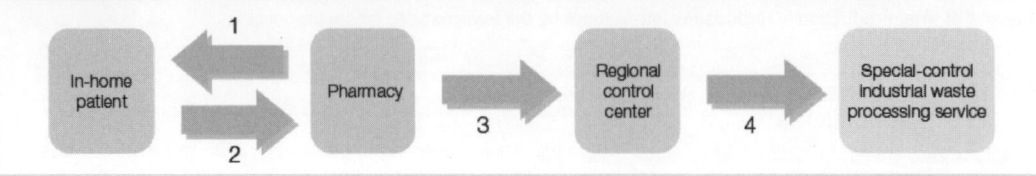

In-home patient → Pharmacy → Regional control center → Special-control industrial waste processing service

http://www2.kankyo.metro.tokyo.jp/kouhou/env/eng/pdf/08.pdf
東京都環境局ホームページ

Glossary

auspices	主催で，賛助で	under the auspices of the company
enacted	（法律などを）制定する，成立させる	
municipality	【名】（地方）自治体，市町村	
syringe	【名】注射器　【他動】注入する	
threatening	脅かすような　　threaten　脅かす	

Expanding your vocabulary

Complete each sentence with the correct form of the most suitable word from the list. 次のリストから適切な単語を選び，正しい形にして文章を完成させなさい．

aggressive 攻撃的な	noncombustible 不燃の
combustible 可燃の	utilization 利用
municipal 地方自治体の	bulky 大きい，かさばる
rechargeable 再充電可能な	designate 指定する

appliance　電気製品 pharmacy　薬局
coordination　調整 vendor　売る人，業者

1. He is responsible for the (　　) of the project.
2. Certain areas are (　　) for special subsidies to attract businesses.
3. The (　　) taxes were high compared to the state taxes.
4. We need some (　　) approaches to reform the current educational system.
5. (　　) substances are able or likely to catch fire and burn.
6. Today's topic is (　　) of alternative and renewable energy sources.
7. The unit runs on (　　) batteries, which last for more than three hours.
8. The house was equipped with many kitchen (　　).
9. Separate the garbage into burnable and (　　) items.
10. We are trying to evaluate competing technologies and products from multiple (　　).
11. You must avoid traveling with (　　) and awkward baggage.
12. He went to the (　　) to fill the prescription from his doctor.

Reading the text for details

Different types of visual aids are used to effectively present the information in the text.
  Data on how much waste was handled by Tokyo in fiscal 2003 (**pie chart**)
  Changes in the volume of waste disposed over time (**bar graph**)
  Process of how waste is handled by Tokyo (**flow chart**)

Answer the following questions based on the visual aids and the text.　図表と文書を参考に次の質問に答えなさい．

1. How much municipal waste was generated in the 23 wards in Tokyo in 2002?
2. List the kinds of municipal waste collected in Tokyo.
3. When was "the Basic Law for Promotion of a Recycling-based Society" enacted?
4. What does "EPR" stand for?
5. According to the text, what is EPR expected to boost?
6. Under what law are personal computers and compact rechargable batteries designated as products to be recycled?
7. When did collection of used syringes by pharmacies begin in Tokyo?
8. Who took the initiative for collection of used syringes?

Practicing a text feature

グラフや図からできるだけ多くの情報を得てみましょう．

1. Waste Categories （p. 27 上）
   廃棄物を図に従って分類し，分類された項目について例を挙げてください．
   Municipal waste = (A.   ), (B.   ), (C.   )
   Industrial waste = (D.   ), (E.   )

   A. = (   )   D. = (   )
   B. = (   )   E. = (   )
   C. = (   )

2. Volume of municipal waste by type in Tokyo (FY2003) （p. 27 下）
   A. ゴミの種類について，それぞれ日本語では何と呼んでいるでしょう？（例：不燃ゴミ，可燃ゴミ，大型ゴミなど）　辞書を引かずに数字情報から類推してみましょう．
   Combustible waste = (a.   )
   Non-combustible waste = (b.   )
   Recyclable waste = (c.   )
   Bulky waste = (d.   )
   Waste brought in directly = (e.   )

   B. Combustible waste の量は，何トンですか？
   　（　　　）トン

3. Trends in waste volume in Tokyo (including recyclable waste); Trends in final disposal volume municipal waste in Tokyo （p. 28）
   A. 2つの棒グラフはそれぞれ，何の推移を表していますか？

   B. 上のグラフからどのようなことが読み取れますか？

   C. 下のグラフからどのようなことが読み取れますか？

   D. BとCから得られた情報を総合すると，どのようなことが類推できますか？

4. FY2003 Flow of municipal waste in Tokyo （p. 29）

図の数字情報を読み取り，次の 3 つの等式を完成させなさい．

(X. Total volume of resource convention) = (a.   ) + (b.   ) + (c.   )

(Y. Volume of final treatment) = (d.   ) + (e.   )

(Z. Volume of waste reduction) = (f.   ) − (g.   ) − (h.   )

X, Y, Z が，それぞれ何を意味しているか，類推してみましょう．
X. (   )
Y. (   )
Z. (   )

5. Collection of Syringes by Pharmacies（p. 30）
   A. 患者が，注射針を薬局で購入し自宅使用する場合の，注射針購入から使用済み注射針回収までの経路を，図から類推しましょう．

   B. 図の上の 1 − 4 のセンテンスは，図 1 − 4 のプロセス（矢印）に対応しています．センテンスを読み，
      a. A. で類推した内容と一致していましたか？

      b. センテンスから得られた新たな情報にはどのようなものがありますか？

Saying it yourself （CD：トラック 5）

Listen to the CD and then practice reading the following passage with good pronunciation and intonation. Pay particular attention to the reading of the years. Mark the pauses with a slash and underline the strongly accented portions.

Collection of used syringes by pharmacies began in November 2002 under the initiative of the Tokyo Pharmaceutical Association, under the auspices of TMG. Starting in Suginami and Nerima wards, it has expanded since 2003 and a total of 20 wards, 10 cities, and 3 towns carry out the collection of syringes as of the end of FY2004.

英語あれこれノート

　ごみと一口にいっても，関連する単語は様々である．また，国によっても呼び方が異なる．数例を挙げたので，参考にされたし．

ごみ収集車	a garbage truck（米），a dustcart（英）
ごみ箱	a garbage can（米），a dustbin（英）
ごみ袋	a trash bag（米），a rubbish bag（英）
ごみ焼却施設	garbage incinerating facilities
ごみ捨て場	a dumping ground

Unit 6

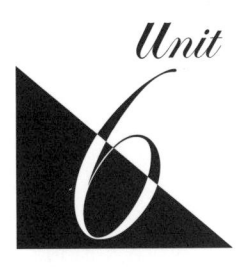

Genre: **Professional organization**
Source: **American Academy of Allergy Asthma and Immunology**

AAAAI（American Academy of Allergy Asthma and Immunology）　米国アレルギー・喘息・免疫学会　　URL▸▸▸ http://www.aaaai.org/

　アメリカ合衆国における，アレルギー・喘息・免疫に関わる最大規模の学会である．学会構成員は，アレルギー学，臨床免疫学ほかの関連学術分野の研究者や専門家からなり，2006年現在，総勢6,300人を越す．定期刊行学術誌として「Journal of Allergy and Clinical Immunology」を発行し，学会ホームページにおいてはアレルギーに関する基本的な情報を掲載しているほか，全米のアレルギーや免疫学の専門家の検索も行うことができる．

日本における食品中のアレルギー物質表示制度

　アレルギー物質を含む食品に関しては，それに起因する健康への悪影響が多く見られ，表示を通じた消費者への情報提供の必要性が高まっていた．しかし，従来の食品に関する表示制度では，その原材料について表示義務が課されない場合等があり，消費者が食品中のアレルギー物質の有無を知るには不十分であった．そのため2002年4月1日，消費者の健康危害の発生を防止する観点から，食品衛生法において，アレルギー物質を含む食品にあってはそれを含む旨の表示を義務付けることとした．

　　　URL▸▸▸ http://www.mhlw.go.jp/english/topics/qa/allergies/index.html

Observing the text as a whole

Look at the following page and think about its PAIL characteristics.　（**PAIL: P** = Purpose　文章の目的，**A** = Audience　文章の対象者，**I** = Information　情報の内容，**L** = Language features　文章の構成形態）

Genre:　　　　　　Explanation and advice about a disease　病気に関する説明と助言
Purpose:　　　　　To inform the public about a disease　人々に病気について情報を与える
Audience:　　　　 General public　一般の人々
Information:　　　Definition, causes, symptoms of a disease　病気の定義，原因，症状
Language features: Question & answer format　質疑応答の形式
　　　　　　　　　　Simple explanations　平易な説明
　　　　　　　　　　Lists of items　項目の列挙
　　　　　　　　　　Pronunciation aids　語句の読みに関する注釈

The American Academy of Allergy, Asthma & Immunology

Food Allergies and Reactions

What are food allergies?

When some people eat certain foods, even a tiny bit, they can have an allergic reaction, such as a rash, runny nose or itchy eyes. Some could even have a more serious reaction that can cause death. That type of reaction is called anaphylaxis (*an-a-fi-LAK-sis*).

A food that causes an allergic reaction is called a food allergen. It's usually the protein part of the food (also called a food protein) that cause the allergic reaction.

Which foods cause allergic reactions?

In children, six foods cause almost all food allergy reactions:

- Milk
- Egg
- Peanuts
- Wheat
- Soy
- Tree nuts (like walnuts and pecans)

Both raw and cooked foods can cause allergic reactions. (Cooking a food does not prevent it from causing an allergic reaction.) Children will often outgrow an allergy to eggs, milk and soy. In adults, four foods cause almost all food allergy reactions:

- Peanuts
- Tree nuts
- Fish
- Shellfish

Who gets food allergies? Can they be stopped?

Once you have food allergies, there are not any medicines that make food allergies go away. If you are allergic to a certain food, the only way to make sure you won't have a reaction is to never taste, touch or even smell the food.

Moms who breast feed their babies might keep the babies from getting food allergies. Another way to keep babies from getting food allergies is to wait to feed them foods that often cause food allergies:

- Try to wait until babies are 6 months old before you give them solid foods. Wait until they are 1 year old before giving them milk and other dairy (like cheese

and yogurt).
- Toddlers should not eat eggs until they are 2 years old.
- Children should not eat peanuts, nuts or fish until they are 3 years old.

Talk to your doctor about a plan for introducing these foods.

How can I tell if I have food allergies?

If you think you are allergic to a food, an allergist/immunologist will do tests to find out which foods you are allergic to.

What are the signs of a food allergy?

Your body could respond in several ways if you are allergic to a certain food:
- Your skin could become red, itchy or develop a rash.
- Your nose could become stuffy or itchy, you might start sneezing, or your eyes could itch and develop tears.
- You might vomit, have stomach cramps or diarrhea.

How dangerous are food allergies?

Food allergies can lead to death. A life-threatening reaction caused by allergy is called *anaphylaxis (an-a-fi-LAK-sis)*. You need to immediately call 9-1-1 if the following happens after you eat something:
- Hoarseness, throat tightness, or a lump in your throat.
- Wheezing, chest tightness or having a hard time breathing.
- Tingling in the hands or feet, lips or scalp.

If you have any of these reactions, call 9-1-1. An anaphylactic reaction moves very quickly and can cause death.

What should I do if I have one or more food allergies?

Avoid the food (or food proteins) you're allergic to. If, for example, you're allergic to milk, avoid milk, yogurt, ice cream and anything that is made with milk. This sounds simple, but food proteins can hide in places you might not expect to find them, most often as ingredients in other foods.

Food labels usually list all the ingredients in any given food. That's why it's a good idea, if you have food allergies, to read the labels. If you see one of your food allergens is listed, don't eat the food. The problem, though, is that a food protein can have more than one name. Different names for some food ingredients appear below:

> Milk proteins:
>
> - Casein, caseinates, rennet casein
> - Lactalbumin, lactalbumin phosphate, lactoglobulin, lactulose
>
> Egg proteins:
>
> - Albumin (also spelled albumen)
> - Meringue or meringue powder
> - These items also may include egg protein: artificial flavors; lecithin; macaroni; marzipan; marshmallows; nougat, and pasta. Read the label of these products very carefully.
>
> If you are allergic to peanuts, avoid the following ingredients:
>
> - Artificial nuts, beer nuts, ground nuts, mixed nuts, monkey nuts, nut pieces
> - Cold pressed, expelled or extruded peanut oil or arachis oil
> - Mandelonas
> - Peanut butter, peanut flour
> - These items may include peanut protein: African, Chinese, Indonesian, Mexican, Thai and Vietnamese dishes; baked goods; candy; chili; egg rolls; enchilada sauce; flavoring; marzipan; nougat, and sunflower seeds.
>
> If you have food allergies, don't be shy about asking restaurants, friends, or anyone else serving you food to list the food's ingredients. Tell them you have food allergies and it's important that you know so that you don't become sick.
>
> Food allergy is a serious condition, but by working with your doctor and avoiding foods, you can stay healthy. Your doctor can answer other questions you might have about food allergies. Visit www.aaaai.org for more educational materials on food allergies.
>
> http://www.aaaai.org/patients/resources/easy_reader/food.pdf
American Academy of Allergy, Asthma & Immunology (AAAAI) ホームページ

Glossary

albumen	albumin と同じ意味
albumin	アルブミン，卵白，（植物の）胚乳
allergen	アレルゲン，アレルギー抗体
allergic	【形】アレルギーの
allergist	アレルギー専門医
allergy	【名】アレルギー
anaphylactic	【形】過敏症の
anaphylaxis	【名】過敏症
casein	カゼイン（牛乳タンパクの一種）
caseinate	カゼイン塩，カゼイン酸
cramp	痙攣，激しい腹痛
enchilada	エンチラーダ（ひき肉を入れたトルティーヤにチリソースをかけたメキシコ料理）．

expel	排出する
extrude	（ものを）押し出す，突き出す
goods	商品
hoarseness	（声の）かすれ
immunologist	免疫学専門医
itch	痒み
itchy	痒い
lactalbumin	ラクトアルブミン（牛乳タンパクの一種）
lactoglobulin	ラクトグロブリン（牛乳タンパクの一種）
lactulose	ラクチュロース（ミルクオリゴ糖）
lecithin	レシチン（リン脂質を含む脂質製品．卵黄や大豆に多く含まれる）
marzipan	マジパン（いったアーモンドと砂糖・卵とを練り合わせたもの）．
meringue	メレンゲ（砂糖と卵白などを混ぜて焼いたもの）．
nougat	ヌガー（糖菓）
outgrow	成長して（悪習・趣味・疾病から）脱却する
pecan	ペカンの堅果（ナッツとして食用）
phosphate	リン酸塩
rennet	レンネット（凝乳酵素を含む物質）
runny	（鼻・目が）粘液を分泌する
scalp	頭皮
shellfish	貝類
sneeze	くしゃみをする
stuffy	（鼻が）詰まった
throat tightness	のどの詰まり
tingling	（体などが）ひりひり（きりきり，ちくちく）する
toddler	よちよち歩きの幼児
vomit	嘔吐する
wheeze	ぜいぜい苦しそうに息をする，息を切らす

Expanding your vocabulary

Complete the following sentences with the most suitable word or phrase from the list below.

a tiny bit	**baked goods**	**dishes**	**peanut butter**	**runny**
anaphylaxis	**breathing**	**itchy**	**restaurants**	**throat**

My friend is allergic to peanuts and therefore must be very careful when eating at (1.   ) that serve Chinese, Thai and Vietnamese (2.   ) that often include peanuts. She must also be careful when buying (3.   ), such as cookies, bread, and cakes. She says that even eating (4.   ) of something containing peanut protein can cause a rash, (5.   ) nose and (6.   ) eyes. She has even been rushed to the hospital due to (7.   ) which can cause death. When this happened, she had a hard time (8.   ) and also felt a tightness in her (9.   ). She says she has gotten used to living with her allergy but is sad that she can never try a (10.   ) and jelly sandwich.

Reading the text for details

Decide whether the following statements are true (T), false (F) or not stated (NS) in the text.

1. Even a very small amount of food can cause an allergic reaction in some people.
2. All allergic reactions are anaphylactic.
3. Most allergic reactions are caused by food proteins.
4. Only six foods cause all allergic reactions.
5. Allergic reactions can be prevented by cooking the food.
6. The shellfish caught in local waters does not tend to cause allergic reactions.
7. Delaying the feeding of foods that cause allergies can help reduce allergic reactions.
8. The patch test is useful for determining whether or not a person has an allergy.
9. Allergic reactions include skin, nose and gastrointestinal symptoms.
10. Food proteins causing allergy are always listed on food labels.

Practicing a text feature

この文書は，各セクションの heading が質問で，セクションの内容が質問に対する答えという質疑応答の形を取っています．

1. 質問に対する一般的な回答（general answer）と，具体的にどうすればよいかという助言の機能を果たしている回答（specific answer）のそれぞれに，異なる色のマーカーでハイライトをつけなさい．
2. 食用蛋白質 milk protein, egg protein, peanut protein は最もアレルギーを起こしやすい物質です．これら3つの物質を含有する食製品およびこれらの製品を避けるためのラベルの見方について，具体的な助言が与えられています．情報を次の表に整理してみましょう．

アレルギーの原因となる食用蛋白質	蛋白質の名称（製品ラベルに用いられている）	蛋白質の含まれている食品

Saying it yourself (CD：トラック6)

Listen to the CD and fill in each blank with the word that you hear. Practice reading the passage aloud.

The summary outlines the system under which (*1.   *) processed foods and food additives are to be labeled. The foods selected for labeling are those which are considered to be health (*2.   *) due to having caused serious allergic (*3.   *) in the past. There are two types of labeling, (*4.   *) and recommended. Foods that must be (*5.   *) are eggs, milk, wheat, (*6.   *) and peanuts. These foods must be given on the food label even when their amounts are very small. Labeling is (*7.   *) for seafood such as shrimp or (*8.   *) and crab and for meats such as beef, chicken and pork. As some people are allergic to (*9.   *) and mushrooms, labeling is also (*10.   *) for these foods.

英語あれこれノート

Many Japanese food names have found their way into the English language. Can you complete the following sentences with the Japanese word in romaji characters?

1. A traditional Japanese breakfast includes (   ) soup.
2. (   ) mushrooms can be used in many kinds of dishes.
3. I love (   ) where we cook thin beef strips with onions and greens and dip them in raw egg to eat them.
4. (   ), which is made from soybeans, is a very healthy source of protein.
5. One of my favorite types of (   ) is the California roll which includes cucumber, crab stick and avocado.
6. Buckwheat noodles, or (   ), is one of my favorite dishes.
7. (   ) is sometimes called Japanese pizza.
8. Our group often goes to a (   ) restaurant because we all love chicken.
9. Instant (   ) can be a very convenient emergency food.

(答えは巻末に)

Try!

Make your own sentence with a Japanese dish that you think would be known by an international audience. Try using it when you next have a chance to talk to someone who is from not Japan.

Unit 7

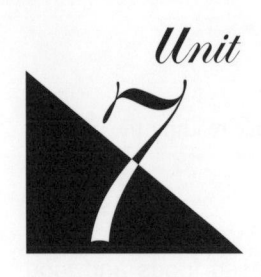

Genre: **News article**
Source: **New York Times**

New York Times

　米国の主力新聞社ニューヨークタイムズ社が発刊する New York Times は，1851 年に創刊され，いまや世界的に有名な米国を代表する日刊新聞である．その紙面には，国内外の政治や経済，健康，科学，スポーツなどに関する「ニュース」，社説や読者からの投稿で構成される「論説」，各種情報に関する「特集記事」などが掲載されている．この新聞の特徴は，多様な意見と豊富な情報を速やかに提供する点である．"中立で公正な新聞" として高い評価を得ており，米国内のみならず世界的にも影響力の強い新聞である．1995 年からはインターネット版が公開されている．
　この章では，健康に関する記事の中から，日本で問題となった小児における抗インフルエンザ薬タミフル®の副作用情報について書かれた記事をとりあげる．薬との因果関係はいまだ明らかにされてはいないが，日本では既に製薬会社に注意喚起の表示が義務づけられている．2006 年 11 月には，米国食品医薬品局 FDA も表示を求める方針を発表している．

Observing the text as a whole

　Look at the following page and think about its PAIL characteristics. （**PAIL: P** = Purpose　文章の目的，**A** = Audience　文章の対象者，**I** = Information　情報の内容，**L** = Language features　文章の構成形態）

Genre:　　　　　　News article ニュース記事
Purpose:　　　　　To inform about news events　起こった出来事を速報する
Audience:　　　　 General public　一般の人々
Information:　　　Problems with the use of an anti-influenza drug　抗インフルエンザ薬に関する問題
Language features: Newspaper reporting style (5W1H)　ニュース報道
　　　　　　　　　　Short paragraphs　短い段落

Childhood Deaths in Japan Bring New Look at Flu Drug

By ANDREW POLLACK

Published: November 18, 2005

The Food and Drug Administration is looking into reports of deaths and abnormal behavior among children in Japan who took the anti-influenza drug Tamiflu, which is being stockpiled by governments around the world for use in a possible flu pandemic.

The agency said that given the available information, it could not conclude that Tamiflu had caused the deaths and other problems. It plans to continue monitor possible complications from the drug for up to two years.

Roche, the company that sells Tamiflu, said that the reports of these problems were rare given that millions of people had used the drug, and that the problems might have been caused by the flu itself.

The issue of Tamiflu's safety in children will be discussed today by an advisory committee to the F.D.A. at a meeting in Gaithersburg, Md. Such a safety review is required one year after a drug receives a patent extension offered to companies that test the safety and effectiveness of their medicines in children.

Seven other drugs will also be discussed at the meeting, but most of the time will be devoted to Tamiflu, also called oseltamivir. While the discussion is not directly related to planning for a pandemic, the F.D.A. said that a better understanding of the safety of Tamiflu for children would be useful in such a situation.

Tamiflu was approved in 1999 in the United States and late in 2000 in Japan. In documents prepared for the meeting, F.D.A. reviewers said 12 children, ages 1 to 16, had died after taking the drug, all of them in Japan. In one document, the reviewers commented on the death of six children ages 2 to 4 who had apparently been healthy before getting the flu. "It is concerning that six young patients died suddenly within one to two days after initiation of oseltamivir therapy," the reviewers wrote.

The documents also said there had been 32 instances of "neuropsychiatric events," 31 of them in Japan, including delirium, abnormal behavior and hallucination.

Two boys, one 12 and one 13, jumped from the second-story windows of their homes after receiving two doses of Tamiflu. Those boys survived, but Japanese news reports have told of two teenagers taking Tamiflu whose death may be attributable to suicide. And an 8-year-old boy had a frightening hallucination and rushed out of his house into the street three hours after his first dose.

There have also been reports of severe skin reactions, in Japan and other countries and in adults as well as children.

One reason so many of the reports are from Japan could be that the drug is used far more widely there than in any other country. Of the 13 million prescriptions written for children worldwide, 11.6 million have been in Japan, according to Roche. That could mean that rare side effects are being seen first in Japan.

But, the F.D.A. said, there may be other reasons. For one, Japanese doctors seem to be more aware of brain inflammation caused by flu itself. That could lead to greater reporting of problems experienced by flu patients, some of whom happen to take Tamiflu.

Roche said that the death rate among children taking Tamiflu was only one in a million and that the rate of death and other problems was no greater than in children with the flu who did not take the drug.

"There is the complicating factor of the disease itself causing these effects," Dr. Joseph Hoffman, a vice president for pharmaceutical development at Roche, said in an interview. He said that in some of the cases of possible side effects, other causes might exist, including other drugs the patients were taking.

Dr. Hoffman also said that one study using data from an insurance company suggested that the use of Tamiflu could reduce the death rate from flu.

http://www.nytimes.com/2005/11/18/health/18tamiflu.html?ex=1165467600&en=d8d01a8d55cb12ee&ei=5070

Copyright © 2005 by The New York Times Co. Reprinted with permission.

Check!

タミフル®（リン酸オセルタミビル）：抗インフルエンザウイルス薬．インフルエンザA型とB型のウイルスのノイラミニダーゼを選択的に阻害し，細胞内で増殖・形成されたウイルスが細胞外に放出されるのを抑制することで，ウイルスの感染・増殖を抑制する．このため，インフルエンザ様症状が発現してから48時間以内に投与を開始する．それ以降の使用では効果は期待できない．タミフル服用後の小児の意識障害や異常行動が報告されているが，その因果関係はいまだ解明されていない．Practicing a text feature の厚生労働省研究班の報告も参照すること．

Expanding your vocabulary

Complete the following sentences with the most suitable word from the list.　空所に入る適切な語をリストから選び，必要なら形を変えて（大文字・小文字，単数・複数の区別，時制など）記入しましょう．

| complication | hallucination | pandemic | reviewer |
| delirium | neuropsychiatric | report | stockpile |

1. Any ( ) of adverse reactions should be immediately sent to the FDA.
2. Several ( ) examined the reports carefully to try to determine the cause of the adverse reaction.
3. As winter approaches, there are fears of a flu ( ) that will affect people around the world.
4. After taking the medicine, the child went into ( ) and became difficult to control.
5. Some countries are ( ) influenza vaccine in anticipation of an epidemic this winter.
6. The drug was monitored for any ( ) that it might cause after an adverse reaction was reported when it was used with an elderly patient.
7. ( ) refer to seeing things that do not exist and can occur as an adverse reaction to a drug.
8. The ( ) problems that were recorded for this drug included hallucinations and abnormal behavior such as attempted suicide.

Reading the text for details

Choose the best way to complete the statements by referring to the news article. Give the number of the paragraph on which you based your response. テキストを参照して，記述に最も合う選択肢を選びましょう．また，どのパラグラフに基いてそう考えたか答えなさい．

1. This news article
   a. describes a new anti-influenza drug.
   b. reports what the Food and Drug Administration is doing.
   c. tells about the stockpiling of a drug.
   d. reports on the influenza situation in Japan.

   Paragraph ( )

2. The FDA
   a. is examining reports of problems with Tamiflu treatment in Japan.
   b. concluded that Tamiflu had caused problems among children in Japan.
   c. said that children should not be given Tamiflu.
   d. found abnormal behavior among children in Japan.

   Paragraph ( )

3. Roche
   a. finds problems with the drug administration.
   b. is monitoring Tamiflu for complications reported in Japan.
   c. reported problems with Tamiflu.
   d. sells the medicine being discussed.

   Paragraph (   )

4. The safety review conducted by the FDA
   a. is done every year for all drugs.
   b. is discussed regularly by the advisory committee.
   c. must be done after a patent extension for children's medicines.
   d. must be conducted at set intervals.

   Paragraph (   )

5. Oseltamivir is
   a. the generic form of Tamiflu.
   b. the medicine for children.
   c. another name for Tamiflu.
   d. not approved by the FDA.

   Paragraph (   )

6. The adverse reactions reported include
   a. pain in the joints.
   b. hallucinations.
   c. breathing problems.
   d. stomachache.

   Paragraph (   )

7. Of the prescriptions written for Tamiflu for children,
   a. about 89% are for children in Japan.
   b. the number is lowest for Japan.
   c. most are for use in the United States.
   d. about 13 million are for children in the United States.

   Paragraph (   )

Practicing a text feature

次のニュース記事は，朝日新聞社が配信しているもので，上の記事に関連する内容を扱っています．下線部の情報をもとに，短い英文ニュース記事を書いてみましょう．

タミフルと異常言動，関連性「なし」 厚労省研究班

2006年10月29日20時38分

A：抗インフルエンザウイルス薬オセルタミビル（商品名タミフル）の服用者が異常言動で死亡した例などが報告されているが，「小児のタミフル服用と異常言動の関連性は認められなかった」という研究結果が厚生労働省の研究班（主任研究者，横田俊平・横浜市立大教授）の調査で分かった．

異常言動は，インフルエンザの合併症として多く発生する脳症の前にも出るとされるが，タミフルの服用が影響しているのか注目されていた．

B：調査は昨年度，全国12都県の小児科医を通して行い，2846件（99.5％が0歳から15歳まで）の回答を得た．発熱後7日間の服薬状況や肺炎や中耳炎の併発，けいれんや意識障害，幻覚やうわごとなどの異常言動があったか答えてもらった．

C：調査対象の患者の9割がタミフルを服用していた．服用した患者の異常言動発生率は11.9％．一方，服用しなかった患者の異常言動の発生率は10.6％だった．統計学的に意味がある差ではなかったという．

医師への調査とは別に，患者の親らにも調査票を配って調べたところ，2545件の回答があった．こちらもタミフル服用による異常言動の発生率の上昇はみられなかった．

厚労省によると，01年の販売開始から今年6月末までに，タミフル服用後に異常言動などで死亡した16歳以下の患者は15人．医薬品による副作用被害に救済金を支給する国の制度に申請した例もあるが，これまでのところ，副作用と認められたケースはない．

D：タミフルは，鳥インフルエンザが変異して起きるとされる新型インフルエンザの治療薬としても期待され，国や自治体が備蓄を進めている．

E：横田教授は「明確な結論を得るにはさらなる検討が必要で今年度も詳細な研究をする」と話す．

http://www.asahi.com/health/news/TKY200610290182.html
asahi.com 2006.10.30付

1. 下線部を短い文に分解して，必要な語彙や言い回しを前の英文記事から探してみましょう．

A
  a. 抗インフルエンザウイルス薬オセルタミビル（商品名タミフル）の服用者が異常言動で死亡した例が報告されている

  b. 「小児のタミフル服用と異常言動の関連性は認められなかった」

  c. ～という研究結果が厚生労働省の研究班（主任研究者，横田俊平・横浜市立大教授）の調査で分かった．

B
  d. 調査は昨年度，全国12都県の小児科医を通して行った．

  e. 2846件（99.5%が0歳から15歳まで）の回答を得た．

C
  f. 服用した患者の異常言動発生率は11.9%．一方，服用しなかった患者の異常言動の発生率は10.6%だった．統計学的に意味がある差ではなかったという．

D
  g. タミフルは，鳥インフルエンザが変異して起きるとされる新型インフルエンザの治療薬として期待されている．

  h. 国や自治体がタミフルの備蓄を進めている．

E
  i. 横田教授は～と話している．

  j. 「明確な結論を得るにはさらなる検討が必要だ」「今年度も詳細な研究をする」

2. A～Eの短文を繋ぎ合わせて，短い英文ニュース記事にしてみましょう（下線部の直訳でなくてもかまいません）．

Saying it yourself （CD：トラック7）

Let's try to practice giving the information from the news article as a news broadcast. Listen to the CD then practice saying the passage yourself.

Announcer: And the next report is about some shocking reports of deaths and abnormal behavior among children in Japan who had taken Tamiflu, an anti-influenza drug. This is the drug that many countries are stockpiling in anticipation of a flu pandemic. The Food and Drug Administration announced today that they are looking into reports of 12 children aged 1 to 16 years who died after being given Tamiflu. They have not yet reached a conclusion as to whether or not the drug was the cause of these deaths. Tamiflu is marketed by Roche. Dr. Joseph Hoffman, vice president for pharmaceutical development at Roche, said that there may have been side effects from other drugs involved. He stated that insurance company data shows that Tamiflu can reduce the number of deaths from flu. He also noted that almost 90% of the some 13 million prescriptions of Tamiflu for children are written in Japan.

英語あれこれノート

Online dictionaries and references can be very helpful. Here are some particularly useful sites:

OneLook Dictionary Search URL▸▸▸ http://www.onelook.com/

Type in a word or a part of a word and it will search more than 900 dictionaries and references for information on it. Some of the dictionaries (e.g. *Merriam-Webster* and *American Heritage*) will pronounce the word for you. This is a great way to practice your pronunciation.

Wikipedia URL▸▸▸ http://en.wikipedia.org/wiki/WIKIPEDIA

As this site is mostly written by volunteers, its reliability has been questioned. However, the respected journal *Nature* conducted a study comparing it with an established encyclopedia and declared it to be quite reliable (http://www.nature.com/nature/journal/v438/n7070/full/438900a.html). This is reported in Japanese at the following site: http://japan.cnet.com/news/media/story/0,2000056023,20093147,00.htm

Unit 8

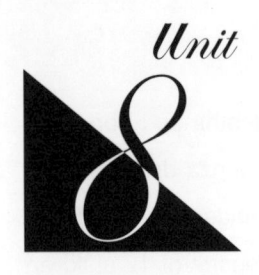

Genre: **Fact sheet**
Source: **Centers for Disease Control and Prevention**

CDC（Centers for Disease Control and Prevention） 疾病管理予防センター

URL▸▸▸ http://www.cdc.gov

　米国保健社会福祉省所管の感染症対策の総合研究所で，医師，薬剤師，獣医師，看護士，農学者，気象学者，微生物学者，細菌学者など多種多様な職員が働いている．このセンターから発表される感染予防や伝搬制御のためのガイドラインは，グローバルスタンダードとみなされるほど影響力がある．CDC のホームページ（http://www.cdc.gov/）は，感染症や伝染病に関する情報のみならず，旅行者向けの情報，遺伝学，環境と健康，虐待や暴力問題など，膨大な数の情報を発信している．

　この章では CDC のホームページから，鳥インフルエンザに関する情報を取り上げる．鳥インフルエンザウイルスのいくつかの亜型は，ヒトへ感染することが確認されている．1997 年の香港 H5N1 型の事例では，一般的なヒトインフルエンザと同様の症状である発熱や咳などから，多臓器不全に至る重症なものまで，様々な症状が報告されている．現在，ヒトにおける鳥インフルエンザがインフルエンザの世界的流行を引き起こす危険性が懸念されている．

Observing the text as a whole

　Look at the following page and think about its PAIL characteristics. （**PAIL: P** = Purpose 文章の目的, **A** = Audience 文章の対象者, **I** = Information 情報の内容, **L** = Language features 文章の構成形態）

Genre:	Fact sheet from government organization　政府機関発行の事実記録
Purpose:	To provide general information about a disease　病気の概要の情報を提供
Audience:	General public　一般の人々
Information:	Avian influenza　鳥インフルエンザ
Language features:	Paragraphs　段落構成
	Technical terms　専門用語の使用

Key Facts About Avian Influenza (Bird Flu) and Avian Influenza A (H5N1) Virus

Avian Influenza (Bird Flu)

Avian influenza in birds

Avian influenza is an infection caused by avian (bird) influenza (flu) viruses. These influenza viruses occur naturally among birds. Wild birds worldwide carry the viruses in their intestines, but usually do not get sick from them. However, avian influenza is very contagious among birds and can make some domesticated birds, including chickens, ducks, and turkeys, very sick and kill them.

Infected birds shed influenza virus in their saliva, nasal secretions, and feces. Susceptible birds become infected when they have contact with contaminated secretions or excretions or with surfaces that are contaminated with secretions or excretions from infected birds. Domesticated birds may become infected with avian influenza virus through direct contact with infected waterfowl or other infected poultry, or through contact with surfaces (such as dirt or cages) or materials (such as water or feed) that have been contaminated with the virus.

Infection with avian influenza viruses in domestic poultry causes two main forms of disease that are distinguished by low and high extremes of virulence. The "low pathogenic" form may go undetected and usually causes only mild symptoms (such as ruffled feathers and a drop in egg production). However, the highly pathogenic form spreads more rapidly through flocks of poultry. This form may cause disease that affects multiple internal organs and has a mortality rate that can reach 90-100% often within 48 hours.

Human infection with avian influenza viruses

There are many different subtypes of type A influenza viruses. These subtypes differ because of changes in certain proteins on the surface of the influenza A virus (hemagglutinin [HA] and neuraminidase [NA] proteins). There are 16 known HA subtypes and 9 known NA subtypes of influenza A viruses. Many different combinations of HA and NA proteins are possible. Each combination represents a different subtype. All known subtypes of influenza A viruses can be found in birds.

Usually, "avian influenza virus" refers to influenza A viruses found chiefly in birds, but infections with these viruses can occur in humans. The risk from avian influenza is generally low to most people, because the viruses do not usually infect humans. However, confirmed cases of human infection from several subtypes of avian influenza infection have been reported since 1997. Most cases of avian influenza infection in humans have resulted from contact with infected poultry (e.g., domesticated chicken, ducks, and turkeys) or surfaces contaminated with secretion/excretions from infected birds. The spread of avian influenza viruses from one ill person to another has been reported very rarely, and transmission has not been observed to continue beyond one person.

"Human influenza virus" usually refers to those subtypes that spread widely among humans. There are only three known A subtypes of influenza viruses (H1N1, H1N2, and H3N2) currently circulating among humans. It is likely that some genetic parts of current human influenza A viruses came from birds originally. Influenza A viruses are constantly changing, and they might adapt over time to infect and spread among humans.

During an outbreak of avian influenza among poultry, there is a possible risk to people who have contact with infected birds or surfaces that have been contaminated with secretions or excretions from infected birds.

Symptoms of avian influenza in humans have ranged from typical human influenza-like symptoms (e.g., fever, cough, sore throat, and muscle aches) to eye infections, pneumonia, severe respiratory diseases (such as acute respiratory distress), and other severe and life-threatening complications. The symptoms of avian influenza may depend on which virus caused the infection.

Studies done in laboratories suggest that some of the prescription medicines approved in the United States for human influenza viruses should work in treating avian influenza infection in humans. However, influenza viruses can become resistant to these drugs, so these medications may not always work. Additional studies are needed to demonstrate the effectiveness of these medicines.

Page last modified February 7, 2006

http://www.cdc.gov/flu/avian/gen-info/facts.htm

Glossary

domesticated	（動植物などを）環境に適応させる
feces	糞便
hemagglutinin	血球凝集素

intestine	腸
mortality rate	死亡率
neuraminidase	ノイラミニダーゼ（ウイルスの表面に存在する糖蛋白で，増殖したウイルスが宿主細胞から遊離する時に働く酵素）
pneumonia	肺炎
ruffled	羽が逆立っている
saliva	唾液
subtype	亜型，サブタイプ
waterfowl	水鳥

Expanding your vocabulary

Complete the following sentences with the most suitable word from the list. 空所に入る適切な語をリストから選び，必要なら形を変えて（大文字・小文字，単数・複数の区別，時制など）記入しましょう．

contagious	**feces**	**intestine**	**pathogenic**	**undetected**
excretion	**influenza**	**nasal**	**saliva**	**virulence**

1. The (　　　) extending from the stomach to the anus are where nutrients are absorbed into the body.
2. Despite various examinations, the cause of her illness remained (　　　).
3. The digestion process begins when (　　　) in the mouth comes into contact with starches.
4. A (　　　) disease can spread quickly from one person to another.
5. The (　　　) are the solid matter discharged from the anus.
6. (　　　) is an acute viral infection in which the patient suffers from fever and inflammation of the respiratory tract.
7. Doctors warned the health officials about the extreme (　　　) of the new disease.
8. (　　　) sprays are used to treat stuffed or runny noses.
9. The (　　　) virus causing the disease was identified by the research team.
10. (　　　), or waste matter, from a living organism include urine and sweat.

Try!

Write a sentence of your own using a word or phrase that you learned in this lesson.

Reading the text for details (CD：トラック 17)

Listen to the CD reading of the text. After you have listened to it once, listen to it again but this time, try shadowing the reader. Practice this two or three times. Complete the following summary with the best word or phrase from the text.

Avian influenza, also known as (*1.*   ), is caused by virus. It is carried by wild birds which usually do not become ill with it. However, the virus is (*2.*   ) among birds. (*3.*   ) fowl can become infected if they come into contact with secretions and (*4.*   ) from virus-carrying birds. There are low and high (*5.*   ) types of the disease.. The highly (*6.*   ) form can very quickly kill also all birds in a flock.

Humans can also become infected with some (*7.*   ) of avian influenza. When there is an (*8.*   ) among poultry, people can become infected if they come into contact with (*9.*   ) secretions or excretions. Medicines may not always be effective because influenza viruses can become (*10.*   ) to them.

Practicing a text feature

1. 文中から情報を探し，A virus を分類してみましょう．

- 鳥インフルエンザについて，H 型と N 型の数，H 型と N 型の組み合わせからなる A virus の亜型（subtype）の数，およびその症状に関する情報を探しなさい．
- ヒトのインフルエンザについて，H 型と N 型の数，H 型と N 型の組み合わせからなる A virus の亜型（subtype）の数，およびその症状に関する情報を探しなさい．

Subtypes of A Virus and the Associated Symptoms

	Number of H(A) subtypes	Number of N(A) subtypes	Number of combination of H(A) and N(A) subtypes	Typical symptoms	
Avian influenza virus	a.	b.	c.	d.	e.
				f.	g.
Human influenza virus	h.	i.	j.	k.	

2. 表を見て，鳥インフルエンザとヒトのインフルエンザの違いを考えてみましょう．

3. 鳥インフルエンザが人間に感染するとどのようなことが起こるでしょう？

Saying it yourself （CD：トラック8）

Listen to the reading of the first paragraph of the text. Mark each pause with a slash (/) and underline or highlight the word stressed the most in each breath group. Note the rising and falling tone at the end of each sentence and where there is a comma.

Avian influenza is an infection caused by avian (bird) influenza (flu) viruses. These influenza viruses occur naturally among birds. Wild birds worldwide carry the viruses in their intestines, but usually do not get sick from them. However, avian influenza is very contagious among birds and can make some domesticated birds, including chickens, ducks, and turkeys, very sick and kill them.

Try!

Choose a section of the text that you would like to practice further. Write the sentences here then mark off the breath groups and the stressed words.

英語あれこれノート

動物が食肉になった場合，名前がかわります．以下の動物と食肉になったときの名前を対応させましょう． （答えは巻末に）

1. chicken   A. beef
2. pig   B. veal
3. cow   C. lamb
4. calf   D. poultry
5. sheep   E. pork

Unit 9

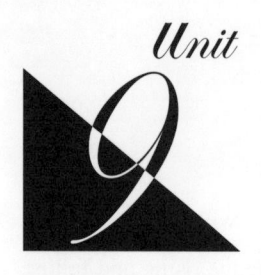

Genre: **Government report**
Source: **Third National Report on Human Exposure to Environmental Chemicals**

CDC（Centers for Disease Control and Prevention） 疾病管理予防センター

URL▸▸▸ http://www.cdc.gov/exposurereport/

米国保険社会福祉省所管の感染症対策総合研究所である．CDCのホームページ（http://www.cdc.gov/）は，感染症や伝染病に関する情報のみならず，環境と健康に関する情報なども発信している．

この章では，CDCにより2005年7月に刊行されたThird National Report on Human Exposure to Environmental Chemicalsを取り上げる．この報告書は，1999年から2002年までの間に，148の環境化学物質に米国民がどれくらい曝露されたかを評価したものである．私たちは，日々多くの化学物質に囲まれて生活しており，これらの化学物質の中には低濃度でも人々の健康に影響を与える物質が存在する．現在，このような化学物質によるリスクの低減や未然防止が重要な課題となっている．

Observing the text as a whole

Look at the following page and think about its PAIL characteristics. （**PAIL: P** = Purpose 文章の目的，**A** = Audience 文章の対象者，**I** = Information 情報の内容，**L** = Language features 文章の構成形態）

Genre:	Government report on environmental chemicals 環境化学物質に関する政府の報告
Purpose:	To report on the exposure of people in the United States to environmental chemicals 米国国民における環境化学物質曝露に関する報告
Audience:	General public 一般の人々
Information:	Description of environmental chemicals 環境化学物質に関する記述
	Data on the extent of exposure to environmental chemicals based on biomonitoring techniques which measure the amounts of these chemicals or their metabolites in human blood or urine 環境化学物質曝露の程度に関するデータ；環境化学物質またはヒトの血液中，尿中代謝産物の量を測定するバイオモニタリング技術を用いて
Language features:	Paragraphs 段落構成
	Many technical terms 専門用語を多数使用
	Topic sentences for paragraphs 段落ごとのトピックセンテンス

Polychlorinated Dibenzo-p-dioxins, Polychlorinated Dibenzofurans, and Coplanar and Mono-ortho-substituted Polychlorinated Biphenyls

General Information

Paragraph 1

Polychlorinated dibenzo-p-dioxins and dibenzofurans (A. _____). They have no known commercial or natural use. Dioxins are primarily produced during the incineration or burning of waste; the bleaching processes used in pulp and paper mills; and the chemical syntheses of trichlorophenoxyacetic acid, hexachlorophene, vinyl chloride, trichlorophenol, and pentachlorophenol. Synthesis and heat-related degradation of polychlorinated biphenyls (PCBs) will produce furan byproducts. As a result of man-made environmental release and contamination, most soil and water samples reveal trace amounts of polychlorinated dibenzo-p-dioxins and dibenzofurans when advanced analytical techniques are applied. Releases from industrial sources have decreased approximately 80% since the 1980s. Today, the largest release of these chemicals occurs as a result of the open burning of household trash and municipal trash, landfill fires, and agricultural and forest fires.

Paragraph 2

The coplanar and mono-ortho-substituted polychlorinated biphenyls (B. _____). Production of PCBs peaked in the early 1970s and was banned in the United States after 1979. Together with the polychlorinated dioxins and furans, these two classes of PCBs are often referred to as "dioxin-like" chemicals because they act through a similar mechanism. In the environment, these dioxin-like chemicals are persistent and usually occur as a mixture of congeners (i.e., compounds that differ by numbers and positions of chlorine atoms attached to the dibenzo-p-dioxin, dibenzofuran, or biphenyl structures). Structural nomenclature is available at http://www.epa.gov/toxteam/pcbid/consistent.htm.

Paragraph 3

People in the general population (C. _____). Breast feeding is a substantial source for infants (Beck et al., 1994). People have also been exposed as a result of industrial accidents (e.g., after an explosion in a factory in Seveso, Italy), the use of accidentally contaminated cooking oils (e.g., as occurred in Yusho in Japan and Yucheng in Taiwan), the spraying of herbicides contaminated with 2,3,7,8-tetrachlorodibenzo-p-dioxin (TCDD, as Agent Orange in Vietnam), and the burning of PCBs contaminated with polychlorinated dibenzofurans, such as in old electrical transformers. Workplace exposures are rare today, and generally recognized standards for external exposure have not been established.

Paragraph 4

Because exposure to these chemicals is from a mixture of varying congeners, the effects (D. _____). However, these four groups of chemicals (polychlorinated dibenzo-p-dioxins, polychlorinated dibenzofurans, and the coplanar and mono-orthosubstituted polychlorinated biphenyls) are considered to act through a similar mechanism to produce toxic effects. These dioxin-like effects are thought to be mediated through an interaction with the aryl hydrocarbon receptor (AhR), particularly the induction of gene expression for cytochromes P450, CYP1A1 and CYP1A2. Dioxins and furans require four lateral chlorine atoms on the dibenzo-p-dioxin or dibenzofuran backbone to bind this receptor. The rank order of interaction with the AhR receptor by degree and position of chlorination is similar for both the dioxin and furan series, with greater effect exhibited with four or five chlorine atoms and with substitution at all four lateral positions. The coplanar polychlorinated biphenyls (unsubstituted at ortho positions) and the mono-ortho-substituted polychlorinated biphenyls (which contain a chlorine atom at one of the ortho positions) can achieve a planar configuration and also interact with the AhR receptor.

Paragraph 5

The variation in the effect on AhR among the dioxin-like chemicals (E. _____). To compare potency, each of these congeners has been assigned a potency value relative to TCDD (toxic equivalency factor [TEF]). When a TEF is multiplied by the concentration of the congener, a toxic equivalency (TEQ) value is obtained. Thus, the dioxin-like toxicity contributed by each of the polychlorinated dibenzo-p-dioxins, dibenzofurans, and coplanar PCBs can then be compared. The sum of all congener TEQs in a specimen (total TEQ) can be used to compare dioxin-like activity among specimens. Many co-planar PCBs have lesser potency, but their concentrations are often much higher than concentrations of TCDD (Kang et al., 1997; Patterson et al., 1994), so their relative contribution to the total TEQ is potentially sizable.

Paragraph 6

Health effects of exposure to dioxins and furans in people (F. _____). Chloracne, biochemical liver test abnormalities, elevated blood lipids, fetal injury, and porphyria cutanea tarda have been reported in many of the studies. In some of these exposures, endocrine, reproductive, and immunologic effects have also been suggested although with varying consistency (Baccarelli et al., 2002; Fierens et al., 2003; Kogevinas, 2001; Halperin et al., 1998; Michalek et al., 1999; Jung et al., 1998; Matsuura et al., 2001; Schnorr et al., 2001; Institute of Medicine, 2003). Congenital anomalies and intrauterine growth retardation were observed in offspring of Yucheng mothers exposed to cooking oil contaminated with electrical oil containing PCBs and dibenzofurans. Background levels of PCBs, and possibly dioxins, have been associated with impaired neurological development in newborns and children (Koopman-Esseboom et al., 1997; Jacobsen and Jacobsen, 1996; Longnecker et al., 2003). A possible dioxin-induced neuropathy may occur in highly exposed adults (Michalek et al., 2001). Many organochlorine-type chemicals, including the dioxins, furans, and PCBs, are also considered to interact with estrogen receptors. Although human studies have yielded inconsistent findings for associations between dioxin exposure and disorders such as endometriosis (Eskenazi et al., 2002; Fierens et al., 2003; Johnson et al., 2001), animal studies have suggested a relationship (Rier and Foster, 2003). The mono-ortho-substituted PCBs (see Table 81) may also interact with estrogen-receptors in addition to their dioxin-like effects, and have been demonstrated to elevate liver enzymes in experimental animals (Parkinson et al., 1983).

Paragraph 7

Carcinogenic, genetic, reproductive, and developmental effects (G. _____). The Institute of Medicine (2003) has determined that human epidemiologic evidence is sufficient for causally linking exposure from herbicides contaminated with TCDD to an increased risk for non-Hodgkin's lymphoma, Hodgkin's lymphoma, chronic lymphocytic leukemia, and soft tissue sarcoma. Generally, the increased risk for these cancers occurs in association with large exposures encountered in contaminated occupational settings or massive unintentional releases. Because of its exceptional potency and because it is the most studied dioxin or furan, TCDD is separately classified by the IARC as a known human carcinogen (Group 1) and by NTP as a known human carcinogen. Other polychlorinated dibenzo-p-dioxins and dibenzofurans have not been studied sufficiently for IARC to determine their carcinogenicity. Information about environmental levels and health effects is available online from ATSDR's Toxicological Profiles at http://www.atsdr.cdc.gov/toxprofiles. The U.S. EPA provides updated exposure and health assessments online at http://www.epa.gov/ncea/pdfs/dioxin.

http://www.cdc.gov/exposurereport/3rd/pdf/thirdreport.pdf

Glossary

aromatic	芳香族（の）
biphenyl	ビフェニル
byproduct	副生物
carcinogen	発癌物質
carcinogenic	発癌性の（ある）　carcino + genic
carcinogenicity	発癌性　carcino + genicity
chlorinate	塩素化する
congener	同属種
congenital	生来の，先天的な
coplanar/planar	共平面の，平面（状）の
cytochrome P450	チトクロム P450（肝の薬物代謝酵素）
dibenzofuran	ジベンゾフラン

dioxin	ダイオキシン
endocrine	内分泌腺，内分泌の　endo + crine
endometriosis	子宮内膜症（子宮内膜やそれに似た組織が子宮内以外の部位に発生し，月経周期に合わせて増殖と剥離を繰り返す）
equivalency	当量
herbicide	除草剤　herb + cide
hexa-	ヘキサ（6を意味する）
immunologic	免疫学の　immuno + logic
ingest	（口から体内に～を）取り込む，摂取する
insulate	防音する，断熱する
intrauterine	子宮内の
lymphocytic	リンパ球
lymphoma	リンパ腫（リンパ節やリンパ組織，またはリンパ球の悪性腫瘍）
neurological	神経学の（に関する・的な）　neuro + logical
neuropathy	神経障害　neuro + pathy
organochlorine	有機塩素
ortho-	オルト（位），o-
penta-	ペンタ（5を意味する）
porphyria	ポルフィリン症（ポルフィリン代謝の先天性代謝異常，体内にポルフィリンおよびその前駆物質が蓄積され，神経症状や皮膚光線過敏症などが発症する）
receptor	受容体
retardation	遅延，精神遅滞
sarcoma	肉腫（非上皮性の悪性腫瘍）
substituted	置換基
toxicity	毒性（度）
tri-	トリ（3を意味する）
unsubstituted	非置換の　un + substituted

Expanding your vocabulary

Complete the following sentences with the most suitable word from the list.　空所に入る適切な語をリストから選び，必要なら形を変えて（大文字・小文字，単数・複数の区別，時制など）記入しましょう．

abnormalities	**contaminants**	**incinerated**	**sizable**
anomaly	**epidemiologic**	**landfill**	**trash**
bleached	**impaired**	**nomenclature**	**unintentional**

1. Carbon dioxide accounts for a (　　) portion of the greenhouse gases.
2. The child was born with a congenital (　　) due to a drug his mother took when she was pregnant.
3. (　　) were discovered in the liver tests, indicating damage from exposure to the chemical.

4. Kansai International Airport is built on a (   ) site.
5. The produce white paper, the pulp must be (   ).
6. (   ) are substances that make something impure.
7. The (   ) is the system for naming things in science.
8. The burning of household (   ) has been banned because it can release harmful chemicals.
9. When waste is (   ), dioxins can be released.
10. Industrial accidents can lead to (   ) release of carcinogens into the environment.
11. (   ) evidence points to the virus as the cause of the disease.
12. Some chemicals can cause (   ) development of the fetus.

Reading the text for details (CD：トラック 18 ～ 24)

The topic sentence of each paragraph is missing the end portion. Based on the information in the paragraph, select which of the following endings best completes the sentence. 各パラグラフのトピックセンテンスの後半部分（本文 A ～ G）が抜けています．最も内容に合う後半部分を下記 1 ～ 7 から選びましょう．

After you have done this, listen to the CD reading of the topic sentences. 次に，トピックセンテンスが録音されている CD を聴きましょう．

(1) due to specific individual congeners are difficult to determine (Masuda et al., 1998; Masuda 2001).

(2) have been observed in many animal studies although species differ dramatically in sensitivity to these chemicals.

(3) belong to the class of chlorinated aromatic hydrocarbon chemicals that once were used as electrical insulating and heat-exchange fluids.

(4) is 10,000-fold, with TCDD and 1,2,3,7,8-pentachlorodibenzo-p-dioxin being the most potent.

(5) are two similar classes of chlorinated aromatic chemicals that are produced as contaminants or byproducts.

(6) have been observed as a result of industrial or accidental exposures involving large quantities of these chemicals.

(7) are exposed primarily through ingestion of foods that are contaminated with polychlorinated dibenzo-p-dioxins and dibenzofurans as a result of the accumulation of these substances in the food chain including high-fat foods, such as dairy products,

of these substances in the food chain including high-fat foods, such as dairy products, eggs, and animal fats, and some fish and wildlife.

Practicing a text feature

各パラグラフごとに次の指示に従って，英語または日本語で情報をまとめなさい．

1. *Paragraph 1*: Dioxin および furan の発生起源についての情報（Hint: 発生起源に関する動詞 = produce）
   Dioxin
   Furan

2. *Paragraph 2*: PCB の歴史に関する情報

3. *Paragraph 3*: 人が polychlorinated dibenzo-p-dioxins や dibenzofurans に曝露，汚染される経路についての情報

4. *Paragraph 4*: Four groups of chemicals が作用するときのメカニズムに関する情報
   A. Four groups of chemicals を挙げなさい．
      a. polychlorinated...
      b. polychlorinated...
      d. coplanar...
      e. mono-orthosubstituted...
   B. a-e に共通のメカニズム

   C. a と b の作用に関するメカニズム

   D. 3 と 4 の作用に関するメカニズム

5. *Paragraph 5*: 汚染物質の毒性比較に関する情報
   TEQ の定義
   PBC の毒性（Hint: 毒性を計る基準は TEQ）

6. *Paragraph 6*: Dioxins および furans が人体におよぼす影響に関する情報
   Confirmed:
   Possibility:

7. *Paragraph 7*: 汚染物質の持つ発がん性，遺伝性，生殖能力および発育に対する影響についての情報

Saying it yourself (CD：トラック 9)

Listen to the CD then practice reading the following topic sentences aloud. Pay particular attention to the pronunciation of the technical terms.

1. Polychlorinated dibenzo-p-dioxins and dibenzofurans are two similar classes of chlorinated aromatic chemicals that are produced as contaminants or byproducts.
2. The coplanar and mono-ortho-substituted polychlorinated biphenyls belong to the class of chlorinated aromatic hydrocarbon chemicals that once were used as electrical insulating and heat-exchange fluids.
3. People in the general population are exposed primarily through ingestion of foods that are contaminated with polychlorinated dibenzo-p-dioxins and dibenzofurans as a result of the accumulation of these substances in the food chain including high-fat foods, such as dairy products, eggs, and animal fats, and some fish and wildlife.
4. Carcinogenic, genetic, reproductive, and developmental effects have been observed in many animal studies although species differ dramatically in sensitivity to these chemicals.

英語あれこれノート

Many technical terms are used in Japanese as *katakana* words. When this occurs, they take on a Japanese pronunciation. When you see a *katakana* word, be careful! Check its pronunciation in English. You will often find it is quite different from what you might expect from the *katakana* form. Can you pronounce the following words with good English pronunciation? カタカナ英語に注意！ 専門用語は外来語（多くは英語由来）のオンパレード．そして，日本式の読み方が定着してしまっています．これら日本式の読みは，英語としては通用しません．外来語の専門用語に出会ったら，必ず，どのように発音するのかをチェックする習慣をつけましょう．次の外来語が，英語ではどのように発音されるのか調べてみましょう．

dibenzofuran	ジベンゾフラン
biphenyl	ビフェニル
ortho-	オルト（位），o-
cytochrome P450	チトクロム P450（肝の薬物代謝酵素）
tri-	トリ（3を意味する）

Unit 10

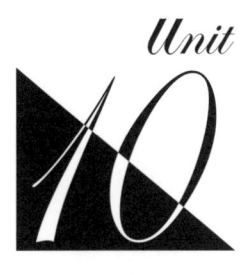

Genre: **Textbook**
Source: **The Anatomy Coloring Book**

The Anatomy Coloring Book

1977 年に発刊された The Anatomy Coloring Book は，「ヒトの身体の構造図に，直接，自分自身で，着色の要点（CN）に従い色分けしながら着色し，人体の器官構造をつくりあげる」という異色の解剖図譜である．塗り絵形式とはいえ，その解剖図は正確で，合わせてその機能が要領よく解説されている．人体の構造と機能を，取り組みやすく，理解しやすく，自己―認識させることを目的として作られた解剖学書である．日本語を始めフランス語，スペイン語，ポルトガル語，イタリア語などに翻訳されている．

この章では，ヒトが生きていく上で最も重要な器官系の 1 つである循環器系（心臓と血管）を取り上げた．色鉛筆片手に，実際にやってみよう！？

Observing the text as a whole

Look at the following page and think about its PAIL characteristics. (**PAIL: P** = Purpose 文章の目的, **A** = Audience 文章の対象者, **I** = Information 情報の内容, **L** = Language features 文章の構成形態)

Genre:	Textbook　教科書
Purpose:	To teach about the circulation system　循環器系について教える
Audience:	Students from junior high and up　中学生以上
Information:	Blood circulation in the human body　ヒトの血液循環
Language features:	Academic style with well-formed paragraphs　整った段落構成を用いた学術用の文体
	Use of formal register　フォーマルな文体
	Illustrations　図解
	Italic fonts　斜体字の使用

VI. CARDIOVASCULAR SYSTEM
SCHEME OF BLOOD CIRCULATION

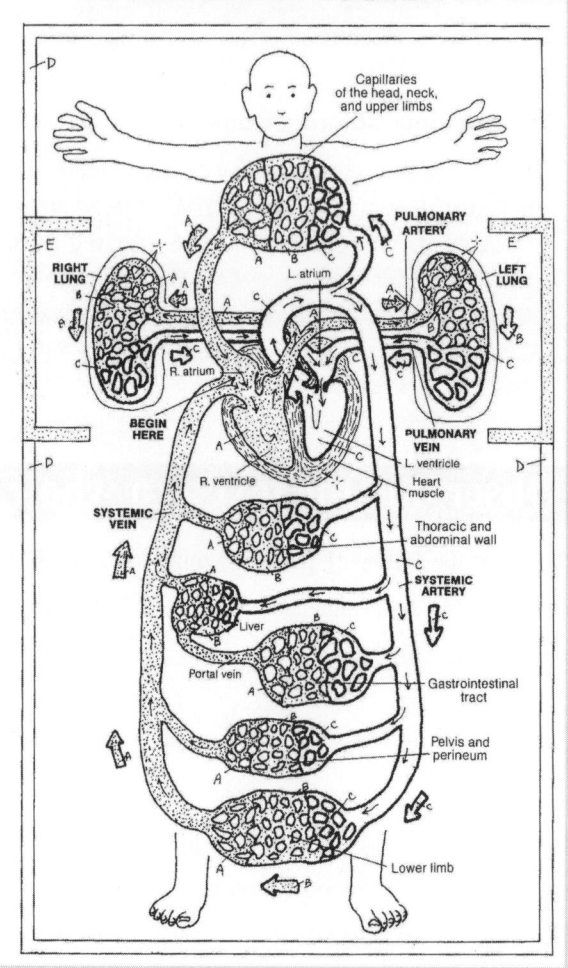

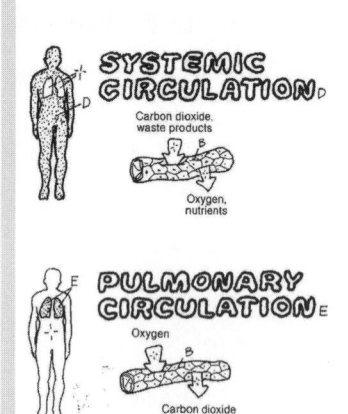

Circulation of blood begins with the heart which pumps blood into arteries and receives blood from veins. Arteries conduct blood away from the heart regardless of the amount of oxygen (oxygenation) in that blood. Veins conduct blood toward the heart, regardless of the degree of oxygenation of the blood. Capillaries are networks of extremely thin-walled vessels throughout the body tissues that permit the exchange of gases and nutrients between the vessel interior (vascular space) and the area external to the vessel (extracellular space). Capillaries receive blood from small arteries and conduct blood to small veins.

There are two circuits of blood flow: (1) the pulmonary circuit, which conveys deoxygenated blood from the right side of the heart to the lungs and freshly oxygenated blood back to the left side of the heart, and (2) the systemic circuit, which conveys oxygenated blood from the left heart to the body tissues and returns deoxygenated blood to the right heart. The color red is used universally for oxygenated blood; the color blue is used for deoxygenated blood.

Clearly, not all arterial blood is oxygenated (in the pulmonary circulation, arteries conduct deoxygenated blood to the lungs), and not all venous blood is deoxygenated (pulmonary veins conduct oxygenated blood to the heart).

Capillary blood is mixed; it is largely oxygenated on the arterial side of the capillary bed, and it is largely deoxygenated on the venous side, as a consequence of delivering oxygen to and picking up carbon dioxide from the tissues it supplies.

One capillary network generally exists between an artery and a vein; an exception is the portal circulation characterized by two capillary sets between artery and vein. The vein between the two networks is the portal vein. Such can be seen between the gastrointestinal tract and the liver.

Page 63 from THE ANATOMY COLORING BOOK, 2nd ed. by Wynn Kapit and Lawrence M.Elson.
Copyright© 1993 by Wynn Kapit and Lawrence M.Elson. Reprinted by permission of Pearson Education, Inc.

Glossary

arterial	動脈の
atrium	心房（心臓の上部にある血液がもどってくる部屋）
bracketing	区分された
capillary	毛細血管（動脈と静脈の間をつなぐ細い血管．組織のなかに入り込み，編み目状にひろがる血管）
deoxygenated blood	静脈血（酸素含量の少ない血液．全身から心臓にもどり肺へ送られる．暗赤色）
deoxygenation	脱酸素化（ここでは，赤血球のヘモグロビンに結合した酸素が解離した状態をさす）
extracellular	細胞外の
gastrointestinal	消化管の，胃腸の
nutrient	栄養物
oxygenated blood	動脈血（酸素含量の多い血液．肺で酸素を取り込んだ後，心臓へもどり，その後全身へ送られる．鮮紅色）
oxygenation	酸素化（ここでは，赤血球のヘモグロビンに酸素が結合した状態をさす）
portal	始まり，発端
pulmonary	肺の
systemic	全身の
transitional	過渡的な
universally	一般に，あまねく
vascular	血管の

Expanding your vocabulary

Give the meaning of the following words by referring to the text. テキストを参照して，次の言葉の意味を英語で答えなさい．

1. arteries
2. veins
3. capillaries
4. the pulmonary circulation
5. the systemic circulation
6. deoxygenated blood
7. oxygenated blood
8. capillary blood
9. a capillary network
10. the portal vein

Reading the text for details

The following are the instructions given in the original textbook material. Do the coloring of the diagram as instructed.

> Use blue for A, purple for B, red for C, and very light colors for D and E. (1) Color the titles for systemic and pulmonary circulation; the two figures; and the borders bracketing the large illustration. Also color purple (representing the transitional state between oxygenation and deoxygenation) the two capillaries, demonstrating the difference between capillary function in the lungs versus the body. (2) Begin in the right atrium of the heart and color the flow of deoxygenated blood (A) into the lungs. After coloring the pulmonary capillary network (B), color the oxygenated blood (C) that re-enters the heart and is pumped into and through the systemic circuit. （以下省略）

Page 63 from THE ANATOMY COLORING BOOK, 2nd ed. by Wynn Kapit and Lawrence M.Elson.
Copyright© 1993 by Wynn Kapit and Lawrence M.Elson. Reprinted by permission of Pearson Education, Inc.

Practicing a text feature

1. 文中の説明に従って血液を3種に分類し，下の空所を埋めて表を完成させなさい．

血液の種類	関連する循環器系の名称	関連する血管の名称
oxygenated blood	the systemic circulation	arteries
	c.	e.
a.	the systemic circulation	f.
	d.	g.
b.	the systemic circulation	(capillary network) arteries and veins
	the portal circulation	h.

2. 本文を読み，図の the portal circulation に当たる部分を○で囲みなさい．
3. 1. の分類に従って，説明文中（第2, 3, 4段落）で oxygenated blood を説明している箇所は赤，a. を説明している箇所は青のハイライトを文中に入れなさい．

Saying it yourself　（CD：トラック 10）

Listen to the CD and fill in each blank with the word that you hear. Practice reading the passage aloud.

The circulation of blood in the body begins in the (1.　　) when oxygenated blood is sent out from the (2.　　) side to the body tissues via the (3.　　). The blood goes to the (4.　　) arteries and then to the (5.　　), which are networks of extremely (6.　　) vessels in the body tissues. This is where (7.　　) and nutrients in the (8.　　) space are exchanged with substances in the (9.　　) space. The (10.　　) blood passes through the small (11.　　) to the large veins to the (12.　　) side of the heart. There it is sent by the (13.　　) circuit to the (14.　　) where it once again becomes (15.　　) and sent to the left side of the heart.

英語あれこれノート

The traditional symbol of the heart ♥ is usually in red to symbolize blood. Its origin is not clear, although there are suggestions that it resembles male and female sexual symbols. The shape is called a cardioid and can be plotted as a graph of $(x^2 + y^2 - 1)^3 = x^2 y^3$ or, in polar form, $r = 1 - \sin(\theta)$.

You have probably seen the I ♥ New York logo or one of its many variations. It is read "I love New York." The logo was designed by Milton Glaser in 1977 for a marketing campaign for New York City. No one expected the logo to become such a hit and Glaser, a professional graphic designer, did the work for free!

URL ▸▸▸ http://en.wikipedia.org/wiki/Heart_(symbol)
http://en.wikipedia.org/wiki/Milton_Glaser
http://en.wikipedia.org/wiki/I_heart_new_york

Unit 11

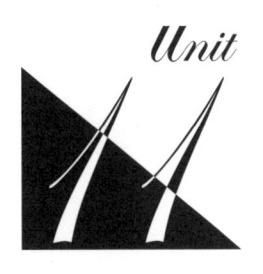

Genre: **Patient Information Sheet**
Source: **American Heart Association**

AHA（American Heart Association） 米国心臓協会

心血管疾患や脳血管疾患の治療や予防，救急医療に関して世界をリードする米国最大の医学学会である．ここでは，これら疾患の治療に関するガイドラインの作成や改訂，予防のための啓蒙活動，心血管疾患による死亡や後遺症を軽減するための専門家や一般向け講習会の開催，学術集会の開催，学術雑誌の刊行などを行っている．

この章では，AHAのホームページに掲載されている一般向け情報の中から，近年，非常に注目されている病態であるメタボリックシンドロームについての項目をとりあげる．メタボリックシンドロームは，肥満，高脂血症，高血圧などの生活習慣を基盤とする疾患が1個人に重積して合併する病態で，動脈硬化のリスクが非常に高いことが知られている．現在，病態やその発症機構，根本的な予防法や治療法の確立などが論争中である．

Observing the text as a whole

Look at the following page and think about its PAIL characteristics. （**PAIL: P** = Purpose 文章の目的, **A** = Audience 文章の対象者, **I** = Information 情報の内容, **L** = Language features 文章の構成形態）

Genre: Patient information sheet 患者用の情報
Purpose: To give patients information about metabolic syndrome メタボリックシンドロームに関する情報を患者に提供する
Audience: Patients and interested general public 患者とこの問題に興味を持つ一般の人々
Information: Definition of disease, criteria for diagnosis, treatment, sources of further information, warning signs of more serious diseases 病気の定義，診断基準，治療，情報源，深刻な病気の兆候
Language features: Question-answer format 質疑応答の形式
Lists (bulleted) 箇条書き
Use of direct address ("you") 二人称を使用しての呼びかけの文体
Explanation of technical terms with details, examples 専門用語を例をあげて詳説

American Heart Association
Learn and Live

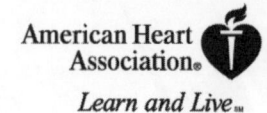

What is Metabolic Syndrome?

This syndrome is a group of metabolic risk factors that exist in one person. There are three root causes of this syndrome:

- overweight/obesity
- physical inactivity
- genetic factors

Metabolic syndrome is a serious health condition. People with it have a higher risk of diseases related to fatty buildups in artery walls. Coronary heart disease, which can lead to heart attack, is an example. Stroke and peripheral vascular disease are other examples.

People with the metabolic syndrome are also more likely to develop type 2 diabetes.

Who has metabolic syndrome?

In recent years this syndrome has become much more common in the United States. About 20 to 25 percent of adult Americans are estimated to have it.

The syndrome is associated with obesity and insulin resistance. Obesity contributes to hypertension, high blood cholesterol, low HDL cholesterol ("good" cholesterol) and hyperglycemia (high blood sugar). Abdominal obesity specially correlates with metabolic risk factors. Metabolic syndrome is considered a clustering of metabolic complications of obesity.

In insulin resistance, the body can't use insulin efficiently. That's a problem because the body needs insulin to convert sugar and starch into energy for daily life and can lead to diabetes.

Some people inherit a tendency toward insulin resistance. In these people, acquired factors (excess body fat and physical inactivity) can trigger insulin resistance and the metabolic syndrome. Most people with insulin resistance have central (abdominal) obesity.

How is the metabolic syndrome diagnosed?

The most current and widely used criteria identify this syndrome by the presence of three or more of these components:

- Central obesity. This is measured by waist circumference:
  - More than 40 inches for men.
  - More than 35 inches for women.
- Fasting blood triglycerides are 150 mg/dL or more.
- Low HDL cholesterol levels:
  - Men — Less than 40 mg/dL
  - Women — Less than 50 mg/dL
- Blood pressure of 130/85 mm Hg or higher.
- Fasting glucose (blood sugar) of 110 mg/dL or more.

What is Metabolic Syndrome? (continued)

What can I do?

People who have the metabolic syndrome can reduce their risk for cardiovascular disease and type 2 diabetes by controlling risk factors. The best way is for them to lose weight and increase their physical activity.

Here are some important steps for patients and their doctors in managing the metabolic syndrome:

- Routinely monitor body weight (especially the index for central obesity). Also watch blood glucose, lipoproteins and blood pressure.
- Treat individual risk factors (hyperlipidemia, high blood pressure and high blood glucose) according to established guidelines.

We need more research to understand how drug therapy might help people with the metabolic syndrome. It's important to focus on the five components of this syndrome to properly manage it.

How can I learn more?

1. Talk to your doctor, nurse or other healthcare professionals. If you have heart disease or have had a stroke, members of your family also may be at higher risk. It's very important for them to make changes now to lower their risk.
2. Call 1-800-AHA-USA1 (1-800-242-8721), or visit americanheart.org to learn more about heart disease.
3. For information on stroke, call 1-888-4-STROKE (1-888-478-7653) or visit us online at StrokeAssociation.org.

We have many other fact sheets and educational booklets to help you make healthier choices to reduce your risk, manage disease or care for a loved one.

Knowledge is power, so *Learn and Live*!

What are the Warning Signs of Heart Attack and Stroke?

Warning Signs of Heart Attack:

Some heart attacks are sudden and intense, but most of them start slowly with mild pain or discomfort with one or more of these symptoms:

- Chest discomfort
- Discomfort in other areas of the upper body
- Shortness of breath with or without chest discomfort
- Other signs including breaking out in a cold sweat, nausea or lightheadedness

Warning Signs of Stroke:

- Sudden weakness or numbness of the face, arm or leg, especially on one side of the body
- Sudden confusion, trouble speaking or understanding
- Sudden trouble seeing in one or both eyes
- Sudden trouble walking, dizziness, loss of balance or coordination
- Sudden, severe headache with no known cause

Learn to recognize a stroke. Time lost is brain lost.

Call 9-1-1... Get to a hospital immediately if you experience signs of a heart attack or

Do you have questions or comments for your doctor or nurse?

- Take a few minutes to write your own questions for the next time you see your healthcare provider. For example:

How can I reduce my weight?

Can physical activity affect my HDL cholesterol?

Can I reduce my blood pressure without taking medicine?

The statistics in this sheet were up to date at publication. For the latest statistics, see the Heart Disease and Stroke Statistics Update at americanheart.org/statistics.
©1994, 2003, 2004, 2005, American Heart Association.

American Heart Association®

Learn and Live™

http://www.americanheart.org/downloadable/heart/1120833743415WhatIsMetabolicSyndrome.pdf

Reproduced with permission

www.americanheart.org

© 2006, American Heart Association, Inc.

Glossary

abdominal	腹部の（診断基準ではウエスト径とされている）
buildup	発達（ここでは，血管壁に脂肪が沈着し内腔が狭くなる，すなわち動脈硬化のことを意味する）
cardiovascular	心血管の，循環器の
circumference	周辺の長さ，回りの距離
correlate	相関する
criteria	基準
dizziness	めまい
hyperglycemia	高血糖（血中グルコース値が高い状態．空腹時血糖値が 126 mg/100 mL 以上や，随時血糖値が 200 mg/100 mL 以上の状態が継続する場合に糖尿病と診断される．血糖値を下げる唯一のホルモンであるインスリンの産生低下や機能低下により生じる）
hyperlipidemia	高脂血症（血中の中性脂肪やコレステロールが高い状態．中性脂肪 150 mg/100 mL 以上，総コレステロール値が 220 mg/100 mL 以上の場合に高脂血症と診断される）
hypertension	高血圧（最高血圧が 140 mmHg 以上または最低血圧が 90 mmHg 以上の状態が継続して観察される場合に診断される）
inactivity	運動不足
lightheadedness	頭のふらつき，立ちくらみ
lipoprotein	リポ蛋白（中性脂肪やコレステロールは水分の多い血液中にそのままでは溶解しにくいが，アポ蛋白と結合しリポ蛋白となって血液中を流れている）
metabolic	代謝性の（メタボリックシンドロームは代謝症候群とも呼ばれる）
nausea	吐き気，嘔気，悪心
numbness	しびれ
obesity	肥満
overweight	過体重（体重が重すぎる，理想体重を超えている状態．一方，肥満は身体に占める脂肪組織の過剰蓄積状態のこと）
shortness	不足すること　　　shortness of breath　息切れ
triglycerides	中性脂肪，トリグリセリド

Expanding your vocabulary

Here are some symptoms associated with heart disease or stroke. They also appear under other circumstances. Choose the best form of the most suitable word for the sentences below. 空所に入る適切な語をリストから選び，必要なら形を変えて（大文字・小文字，単数・複数の区別，時制など）記入しましょう．

cold sweat	**discomfort**	**lightheadedness**	**nausea**	**shortness of breath**
confusion	**dizziness**	**loss of coordination**	**numbness**	**weakness**

1. Feeling as though she were going to fall, she complained of (　　　).
2. The man had a strong feeling of (　　　) in his legs after the accident.
3. Old people suffering from dementia often seem to be in a state of (　　　).
4. After rushing up the stairs to catch the train, she felt a (　　　).

5. Vertigo, or (   ), is a feeling that everything around you is spinning.
6. While walking along a deserted street at night, she broke into a (   ) on hearing footsteps behind her.
7. Motion sickness when riding a car or an airplane is often accompanied by (   ).
8. After the surgery, she felt a (   ) in her arms and had to undergo rehabilitation to regain her strength.
9. The severe cold caused a loss of feeling, or (   ), of the hands and feet.
10. A disease such as polio can cause paralysis and (   ) of the limbs.

Reading the text for details

Answer the following questions based on the information in the text.

1. What are the causes of the metabolic syndrome?

2. Why is this considered to be a serious condition?

3. What problems does obesity lead to?

4. What happens in insulin resistance?

5. What kinds of blood tests are used to diagnose the metabolic syndrome?

6. What is central obesity?

7. What is the best thing to do for people diagnosed with the metabolic syndrome?

8. Why should a person with the metabolic syndrome tell family members about it?

9. If a person with the metabolic syndrome complains for chest discomfort and breaks out into a cold sweat, what could this indicate?

10. If a person with the metabolic syndrome suddenly has a severe headache which does not seem to have a known cause, what should be suspected?

Practicing a text feature

例にならって患者用のチェックシートを作ってみましょう．

チェック項目	yes	no
1. Is your waist circumference more than 40 inches (men)/35 inches* (women)? * 1 inch = 2.54 cm		
2.		
3.		

Saying it yourself (CD：トラック 11)

Complete the following dialogue based on the information in the text. Listen to the CD to check the dialogue then practice saying it.

Give the people names: Person A:_____ Person B:_____

A: The results from the medical check-up came today.
B: Yeah, so did mine. How were your results?
A: What a shock! The doctor said I have the (1.   ) syndrome!
B: Really?! What does that mean?
A: It means that I have a higher risk for (2.   ) disease and (3.   ).
B: Oh, oh. Why is that?
A: Well, it seems that the artery walls get a lot of (4.   ) buildup. That causes problems with blood flow.
B: Ah, I see. How did the doctor (5.   ) it? Can he see the inside of your arteries?
A: Oh, no. There are several (6.   ) for diagnosing the metabolic syndrome. One is the (7.   ) measurement. Others are the amounts of (8.   ), which are fatty acids, and cholesterol in the blood. The (9.   ) pressure and blood sugar level are also considered.
B: So your blood test results were not good?
A: No, they weren't. My total cholesterol level is high and the low HDL (10.   ) level,

which is the good cholesterol, is too low.

B: How confusing! You need to have low total cholesterol but (*11.*   ) low HDL cholesterol?

A: Yeah. I'm also (*12.*   ) and need to lose about 10 kilograms. On top of all that, my blood pressure is a bit high.

B: How about your blood sugar level?

A: Fortunately, that seems to be OK.

B: (*13.*   ) are you going to do?

A: Well, I need to lose weight. So I've decided to take a walk every morning for about an hour.

B: Can you get up early enough to do that?

A: Well, if I can't, then I'll go for a walk in the evening.

B: You should also think about going on a diet to lose (*14.*   ).

A: That's right. I need to cut down on calories.

B: Do you need to take any medicine?

A: The doctor told me to (*15.*   ) more. I need to go for a check-up in a month. I guess he'll decide what to do then. By the way, how were your results?

B: Fine. I got a clean bill of health!

A: Good for you!

英語あれこれノート

For listening practice, the Web offers many great sites, ranging from those for people trying to learn English to those for people wanting to get the latest news. For English language learners, try the following sites:

Dave's ESL Cafe   http://www.eslcafe.com/

　　Find out about idioms, phrasal verbs and grammar.

Randall's ESL Cyber Listening Lab   http://www.esl-lab.com/

　　Test yourself with the General Listening Quizzes.

If you are interested in listening to more challenging material, try out the Nature Podcasts. The great thing is that they have transcripts so that you can follow the audio and get the details.

URL▸▸▸   http://www.nature.com/podcast/index.html

The following site has a World Heart Day podcast (and transcript) which deals with the topic of this unit.

URL▸▸▸   http://www.nature.com/ncpcardio/podcast/index.html

Unit 12

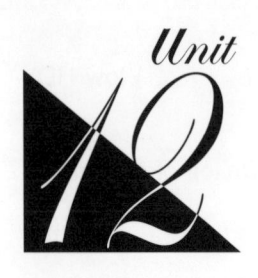

Genre: **Textbook**

Source: **Human Pharmacology: Molecular to Clinical**

Human Pharmacology

　薬が身体のどこにどのように作用し，その結果，身体の機能がどう変化するか，を学ぶ学問が「薬理学」である．薬理学は，薬物療法を適正に行うため，また，新しい薬の開発のための基礎知識となる．薬の作用機序を知るためには，生理学，生化学，分子生物学，遺伝子学などの基礎知識が基盤となる．Human Pharmacology は，分子レベルから臨床的知見まで幅広い情報を収載した薬理学書である．

　この章では，血中の脂質レベルを下げる薬，すなわち，高脂血症治療薬と呼ばれる一連の薬について書かれた章をとりあげる．高脂血症は，心筋梗塞や脳卒中など致死的疾患の発症原因となる動脈硬化（血管壁が固くなり血液循環が悪くなる）の危険因子である．

Observing the text as a whole

Look at the following page and think about its PAIL characteristics. （**PAIL: P** = Purpose　文章の目的，**A** = Audience　文章の対象者，**I** = Information　情報の内容，**L** = Language features　文章の構成形態）

Genre:	Textbook　教科書
Purpose:	To teach students about a subject　学生に学科内容を教える
Audience:	College students majoring in medical sciences　医学を専攻している大学生
Information:	Drugs that lower lipid levels and the mechanism by which this is accomplished　脂肪のレベルを下げる薬品とその効果のメカニズム
Language features:	Formal, academic register　フォーマルな表現，学術文書のスタイル
	Tables and figures　表と図
	Long paragraphs　長いパラグラフ
	Long sentences　長いセンテンス
	Many technical terms　専門用語の多用

Chapter 20
Lipid-lowering Drugs and Atherosclerosis

ABBREVIATIONS	
ACAT	acyl-CoA: cholesterol acyl transferase
acetyl-CoA	acetylcoenzyme A
Apo A	apoprotein A
Apo E	apoprotein E
HDL	high density lipoprotein
HMG-CoA	hydroxy-3-methyl-glutaryl coenzyme A
IDL	intermediate density lipoprotein
LDL	low density lipoprotein
PDGF	platelet-derived growth factor
VLDL	very low density lipoprotein
EGF	epidermal growth factor

MAJOR DRUGS
Bile acid ion-exchange resins
Cholesterol synthesis inhibitors
Fibric acid derivatives
Probucol
Nicotinic acid
Other agents: neomycin and sitosterol

THERAPEUTIC OVERVIEW

Diseases of the heart and blood vessels are the principal causes of death in industrialized countries of the world. In the United States, more people die of such diseases than from cancer or any other illness. Of the deaths resulting from cardiovascular disease, over three-fourths can be attributed to atherosclerosis and its complications. Atherosclerosis is a generalized disease of the arterial tree that usually develops in a symptom-free manner over many years. The most common manifestation of atherosclerosis is coronary heart disease, followed by stroke and peripheral vascular disease. Because it is a slowly developing disorder, treatment must be directed at causative factors and at its prevention rather than its reversal. In primates, studies demonstrate actual reversal of lipid deposits in the arterial wall and a regression of the attendant fibrous tissue. Therefore there is hope for clinical reversal in humans. Coronary artery studies in humans show increases in lumen size with a decrease in blood cholesterol concentration.

Elevated cholesterol concentrations are one of the major contributing factors in the development of atherosclerosis. Cholesterol enters the circulation from two major sources, absorption from food (exogenous pathway) and synthesis by the liver (endogenous pathway). It leaves the circulation when it is taken up by the liver to form bile acids, or taken up by other cells to form steroid hormones or inserted into membranes. When present in excess, it is taken up by fibroblasts and scavenger cells in regenerating tissues, as well as fat cells. <u>(1) Transport of cholesterol within the plasma is by way of lipoprotein particles.</u>

Currently, smoking cessation and lowering plasma concentrations of cholesterol and its associated lipids are the only proven approaches to the prevention of atherosclerosis-related disorders. A variety of clinical studies demonstrate the feasibility of lowering cholesterol with diet and drugs such as niacin, clifibrate, bile-acid binding resins, gemfibrozil and lovastatin (Figure 20-1). Two classical clinical trials show a (2) reduction in total cholesterol and low density lipoprotein and elevation in high density lipoprotein fractions to be clearly associated with a reduced incidence of coronary artery event rates (angina, myocardial infarction, coronary bypass surgery needs, or positive treadmill testing.) In general, for every percentage point that the cholesterol concentration is lowered, a 2% lowering of the risk of coronary heart disease occurs.

The metabolism of cholesterol and fatty acids and their associated lipid transport particles (the lipoproteins), occurs in the gut, liver, and the peripheral tissues. Drugs that alter cholesterol concentrations act, for the most part, by altering the kinetics of one or more parts of the metabolic cycle. Production and secretion of bile formed from cholesterol by liver cells or hepatocytes is necessary for the emulsification of dietary fat and cholesterol before absorption. The majority of the secreted bile is reabsorbed during the digestive process and recycled, but approximately one-third is lost in the stool. (3) Interruption of this cycle by bile-acid binding resins such as cholestyramine, colestipol, and the antibiotic neomycin, results in reduced gastrointestinal (GI) absorption of cholesterol and dietary fats. The prevention of the reabsorption of bile acids has the secondary effect of causing the hepatocyte to synthesize increased amounts of bile. Because cholesterol is the necessary precursor for bile formation, the increased cholesterol utilization reduces the total body pool of cholesterol (4) by promoting an increase in certain receptors and subsequent removal of the fraction that

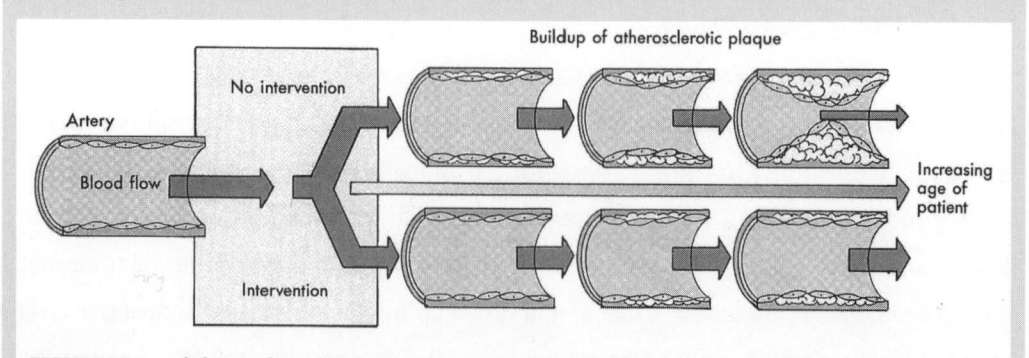

FIGURE 20-1 Atherosclerosis prevention. Intervention (treatment) involves (1) diet to decrease cholesterol and lipids, (2) cessation of smoking, (3) drugs to reduce plasma cholesterol, (4) control of blood pressure, and (5) control of diabetes (see text).

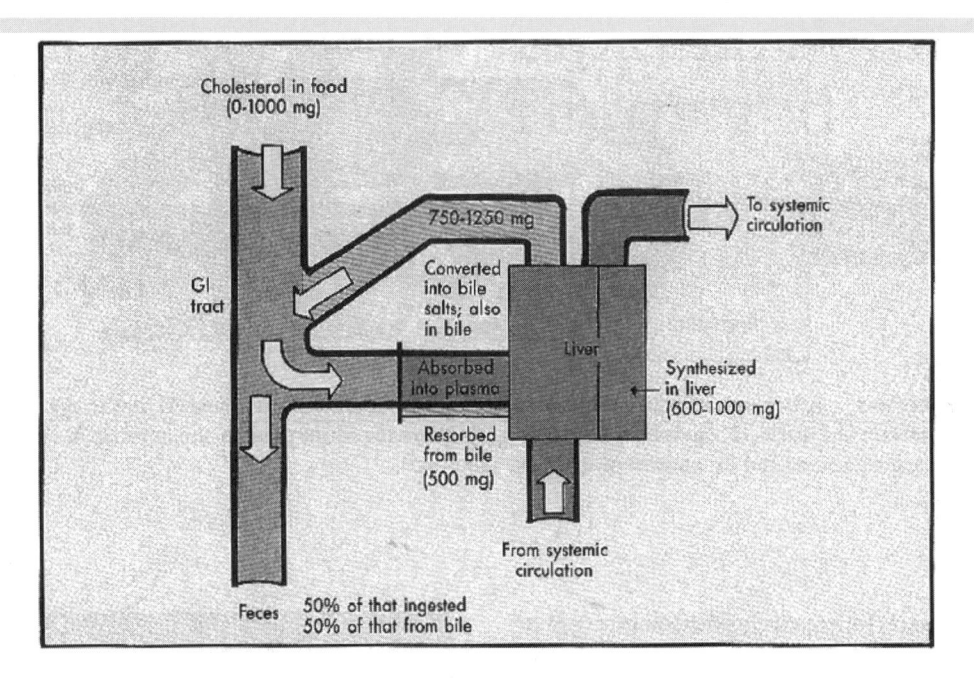

FIGURE 20-2 Total body balance of cholesterol, showing input by ingestion and liver synthesis output by nonabsorption into feces, conversion into bile salts, delivery in bile salts to smal intestine, partial reabsorption from bile, and delivery as lipoproteins into systemic circulation Quantities shown are approximate daily amounts.

binds to these receptors.

Therapeutic uses of lipid-lowering drugs are summarized in the box.

THERAPEUTIC OVERVIEW

ANTILIPID DRUGS

Goal: prevention of myocardial infraction and other atherosclerotic disorders such as stroke and peripheral vascular disease

Approach: prophylactic use to reduce formation of atherosclerotic plaque and subsequent narrowing of lumen in cardiac arteries

Primary risk factors:

  High blood cholesterol and certain lipids

  High blood pressure

  Smoking

  Overweight

  Sedentary lifestyle

Lemuel B. Wingard, Theodore M. Brody, Joseph Larner, Arnold Schwartz, *Human Pharmacology (2nd edtition)*, Mosby Year Book (1991)

Glossary

angina	狭心症（心臓の冠動脈が狭窄することで，それ以降の血液循環が悪くなり，心筋細胞に酸素不足が生じている状態）
arterial	動脈の
atherosclerosis	粥状動脈硬化（血管壁に脂質が沈着したタイプの動脈硬化）
cardiovascular	心臓血管の
causative	原因となる
cessation	中止，中断，休止，停止
cholesterol synthesis inhibitors	コレステロール合成阻害薬（HMG-CoA 還元酵素阻害薬のことをさす）
coronary	冠血管の
dietary	ダイエットの，食餌［食事］療法の
digestive	消化の，消化を助ける
elevate	上昇させる
emulsification	乳状［乳剤］化，乳化（作用）
endogenous	内因性の
exogenous	外因性の
feasibility	実行可能な
fibric acid derivatives	フィブラート系（核内受容体 PPAR α 活性化を介して主として中性脂肪を低下させる）
fibroblast	線維芽細胞（膠原線維や弾性線維を生成する細胞．動脈硬化病変で増加すると，線維化を生じる）
fibrous	線維性の（膠原線維や弾性線維のことをさす．血管壁の構成成分で，弾力性と強度を保持する）
gastrointestinal	消化管の，胃腸の
generalize	一般化する
hepatocyte	肝細胞，肝実質細胞（肝臓を構成する細胞で，肝臓の代謝機能の中心的な役割を担う細胞）
high density lipoprotein	HDL，高比重リポ蛋白（細胞からコレステロールを引き抜くリポ蛋白．HDL が多いほど長寿といわれている）
industrialize	（〜を）産業［工業］化する
infarction	梗塞（ここでは心筋梗塞のこと．冠動脈が動脈硬化などにより閉塞し，心筋細胞へ酸素や栄養を送ることができなくなったために心筋に壊死が生じた状態）
ion-exchange resins	陰イオン交換樹脂（胆汁酸と結合し腸管からの再吸収を抑制することにより，肝臓のコレステロール需要を高めることで血中のコレステロールを下げる．また，胆汁は腸管からの脂質吸収に必須であるため，吸収が抑制されることも血中脂質が下がる要因となる）
kinetics	反応速度
lipid	脂質（中性脂肪，コレステロール，脂肪酸などの総称）
lipoprotein	リポ蛋白（コレステロールや中性脂肪は，アポ蛋白と結合してリポ蛋白となった状態で血中を流れる．リポ蛋白のうち，コレステロールを運ぶのに重要なリポ蛋白が LDL と HDL である．LDL は細胞にコレステロールを運ぶリポ蛋白で，一般的に LDL は悪玉コレステロールといわれる．一方，HDL は細胞からコレステロールを引き抜くリポ蛋白で，HDL が多いほど長寿といわれている）
low density lipoprotein	LDL，低比重リポ蛋白（細胞にコレステロールを運ぶリポ蛋白．LDL が高いと動脈に脂質がたまりやすいことを意味するため，一般的に悪玉コレステロールといわれる）

lumen	管腔，内腔（ここでは血管の内側の血液が流れる空間のこと）
metabolic	代謝性の
myocardial	心筋細胞
nicotinic acid	ニコチン酸（脂質低下作用の機序の詳細は不明）
neomycin and sitosterol	ネオマイシンとシトステロール（脂質低下作用は，腸管からのコレステロールの吸収抑制と考えられている）
precursor	前駆物質
primate	霊長目の動物
probucol	プロブコール（コレステロール低下作用の機序の詳細は不明．抗酸化作用を併せ持つため抗動脈硬化作用が期待されている）
reabsorb	再び吸収する
regenerate	再生する，再生させる
resin	樹脂（陰イオン交換樹脂は，胆汁酸の小腸からの再吸収を阻害する．その結果，胆汁酸はコレステロールから生成されるため肝臓のコレステロール需要を高めることになる．また，胆汁酸は腸管からの脂質吸収に必須であるため胆汁酸が低下すると脂質吸収が抑制されることになる．これらの結果として血中脂質値が下がる）
scavenger	スカベンジャー（マクロファージが脂質を際限なく取り込むようになった状態をスカベンジャー細胞といい，血管壁での脂質沈着に関与する．脂質を貪食した泡沫細胞となり，粥状動脈硬化病変に存在する）
secrete	分泌する
steroid	（副腎皮質）ステロイド
synthesize	合成する
utilize	利用する

Expanding your vocabulary

Match the beginning and ending of the following sentences.

1. Cardiovascular diseases
2. Atherosclerosis
3. Clinical reversal with lipid-lowering drugs
4. Cholesterol in the body
5. Scavenger cells
6. Lipoproteins
7. Coronary artery problems
8. Clinical trials
9. A precursor
10. An antilipid drug

A. take up cholesterol which can cause the build up of lipid deposits in the arterial wall.
B. is a substance needed to form another substance.
C. are diseases of the heart and the blood vessels.
D. comes from exogenous and endogenous pathways.
E. is used to prevent cardiovascular diseases.
F. can be reduced by lowering total cholesterol and low density lipoprotein levels.

G. can occur with decrease of lipid deposits and regression of fibrous tissue in the arteries.
H. are studies to check the efficacy and safety of drugs and new medical treatments.
I. occurs due to lipid deposits in the arterial wall.
J. are particles that transport lipids, i.e. cholesterol and triglycerides, in blood.

Reading the text for details

Answer the following questions based on the information in the text. Give your answers as complete sentences. 本文を参照して，次の問いに英文で答えなさい．

1. Why is it important to treat atherosclerosis?
2. Why is atherosclerosis difficult to detect?
3. What are the three most common diseases caused by atherosclerosis?
4. Why does there seem to be hope for reversal of the buildup of lipid deposits in the arterial wall?
5. How is cholesterol used in the human body?
6. What is known to definitely prevent atherosclerosis?
7. How do most lipid-lowering drugs work?
8. Where in the human body is cholesterol metabolized?
9. How are antilipid drugs used?
10. How can a person reduce the risk of atherosclerosis-related diseases?

Practicing a text feature

For this text, let us consider how to ask questions. Knowing what you do not know and knowing how to learn about it is a very important part of academic life. How would you ask the following questions in English? このユニットの内容を理解するために必要な背景知識について，薬学の専門の先生に尋ねてみました．研究生活においては，常に，「自分が何を知らないか」「知識を得るためにはどうすればよいか」を問い続けなければなりません．下の質疑応答から背景知識を得るだけでなく，質問の仕方についても考えてみてください．そして，日本語による下の質問の文を英語ではどのように言えばよいかを考えてみてください．

Q1：*(1.) Transport of cholesterol within the plasma is by way of lipoprotein particles* とありますが，これはどういうことを意味しますか？

英語：

A1：脂質は油ですので，水である血液中にはミセルとなって，あたかも解けたように存在します（牛乳も同じ）．つまり，脂質はリポ蛋白となって血液中をながれています．リポ蛋白とは，脂質とアポ蛋白などからなるミセルのことです．コレステロールは，リポ蛋白によって運ばれます．

Q2：(2.) reduction in total cholesterol and low density lipoprotein and elevation in high density lipoprotein fractions とありますが，low density lipoprotein, high density lipoprotein とは何ですか？
英語：

A2：リポ蛋白には数種類あって（脂質の存在比率が違うもの），そのうちのコレステロールを運ぶのに重要なリポ蛋白が low density lipoprotein (LDL) と high density lipoprotein (HDL) です．LDL は細胞にコレステロールを運ぶリポ蛋白，HDL は細胞からコレステロールを引き抜くリポ蛋白です．一般的には LDL が悪玉コレステロールといわれるもので，HDL が多いほど長寿といわれています．

Q3：(3.) interruption of this cycle とありますが，this cycle とは，"The majority of the secreted bile is reabsorbed during the digestive process and recycled" の process のことですか？
英語：

A3：そうです．胆汁（胆汁酸）は肝臓で作られ胆嚢で濃縮された後，腸管に分泌されます．分泌された胆汁の一部は，腸管で再吸収され再利用されます．この過程を腸肝循環といいます（Fig. 20-2 参照）．陰イオン交換樹脂のような薬物は，胆汁中の胆汁酸と結合し腸管からの再吸収を抑制します．胆汁酸は腸管からの脂質吸収に必須であるため，胆汁酸が低下すると脂質吸収が抑制され，結果，血中の脂質値が下がります．また，次の文章にあるように，胆汁酸はコステロールから生成されるため，肝臓のコレステロール需要を高めることになり，結果的に血中コレステロールが下がります．

Q4：(4.) by promoting an increase in certain receptors and subsequent removal of the fraction that binds to these receptors とありますが，ロジックがよくわかりません．
英語：

A4：確かに難しいですね．コレステロールの低下は，代償的に肝臓のコレステロール受容体，正確には LDL 受容体の数が増えることにつながります．

Saying it yourself (CD：トラック 12)

Practice reading the following section of the text. In preparing to read it, put in slashes to indicate the pauses and highlight the words that you plan to emphasize. Listen carefully for the stress patterns of the individual words, especially the technical terms.

Getting accustomed to listening to long, technical sentences can help you listen to formal academic lectures. Actually the lectures should be easier to listen to because there is likely to be more repetition. You can try listening to the NIH (National Institutes of Health, USA) podcasts and audio reports

http://www.nih.gov/news/radio/nihpodcast.htm

Previous podcasts are archived at

http://www.nih.gov/news/radio/nihpodcastarchive.htm

The metabolism of cholesterol and fatty acids and their associated lipid transport particles (the lipoproteins) occurs in the gut, liver, and the peripheral tissues. Drugs that alter cholesterol concentrations act, for the most part, by altering the kinetics of one or more parts of the metabolic cycle. Production and secretion of bile formed from cholesterol by liver cells or hepatocytes is necessary for the emulsification of dietary fat and cholesterol before absorption. The majority of the secreted bile is reabsorbed during the digestive process and recycled, but approximately one-third is lost in the stool. Interruption of this cycle by bile-acid binding resins such as cholestyramine, colestipol, and the antibiotic neomycin, results in reduced gastrointestinal (GI) absorption of cholesterol and dietary fats. The prevention of the reabsorption of bile acids has the secondary effect of causing the hepatocyte to synthesize increased amounts of bile. Because cholesterol is the necessary precursor for bile formation, the increased cholesterol utilization reduces the total body pool of cholesterol by promoting an increase in certain receptors and subsequent removal of the fraction that binds to these receptors.

英語あれこれノート

医療情報を収集するためのウェブサイトの紹介

1) RxList

　　URL▸▸▸ http://www.rxlist.com/

　医薬品の基本的な情報を無料で収集できるサイト．化学構造，効能・効果，投与量・投与方法をはじめ，副作用，薬物相互作用，patient information 患者への情報提供（病気に関する説明）などが収集できる．検索は，一般名でも商品名（brand name および generic name）でも可能．

2) Drugs.com

　　URL▸▸▸ http://www.drugs.com/

　医薬品の基本情報を無料で収集できるサイト．一般向け情報として医薬品の基本情報が掲載されており，病気についての解説もある．また，専門家向け情報の中には，ジェネリック医薬品についての情報が掲載されている．

3) US Food and Drug Administration（FDA）の Drug Information

　　URL▸▸▸ http://www.fda.gov/cder/drug/default.htm

　米国食品医薬品局の医薬品に関する情報サイト．米国で承認されている医薬品についての情報が無料で収集できる．ここでは，処方箋薬のみならず，大衆医薬品（OTC 薬）についての情報も公開されている．

4) The Merck Manuals online medical library for healthcare professionals

　　URL▸▸▸ http://www.merck.com/mmpe/index.html

　米国の製薬企業メルク社が運営する医療従事者向けサイト．病気についての一般的な情報をはじめ，治療法や薬に関する情報を無料で収集できる．一般向けサイトとして，The Merck Manual of Medical Information-Home Edition　http://www.merck.com/mmhe/index.html がある．

5) MedicineNet.com

　　URL▸▸▸ http://www.medicinenet.com/script/main/hp.asp

　病気について，その症状や日頃注意すべきサイン，病気の治療方法やその予防法などが，一般向けに解りやすく説明されている健康サイト．薬について，その効能や使用方法，副作用や飲み合わせの注意などに関する情報も掲載されている．

Unit 13

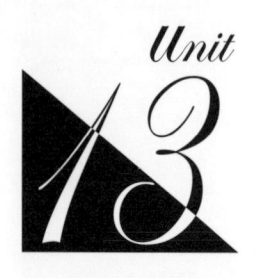

Genre: **Position statement**
Source: **Diabetes Care**

Diabetes Care

　Diabetes Care は，米国糖尿病学会（American Diabetes Association, ADA）が定期刊行する学術雑誌の 1 つである．医師などの臨床家を対象として，糖尿病についての知識を高め，より良い治療を行うための情報を掲載する専門誌である．Diabetes Care には，糖尿病の治療法，疫学調査，救急治療，病態生理，合併症などについて書かれた一般論文，速報論文，総説などが掲載されている（下記参考欄参照）．ADA は 2002 年 1 月 Diabetes Care 増刊号に，糖尿病に対する診療ガイドラインを発表した．この章では，糖尿病やその合併症の治療や予防のための食餌療法の基本方針に関する勧告をとりあげる．

　各種の医学会は，それぞれの疾患に対する診療ガイドラインを作成し公開している．診療ガイドラインとは，予防から診断，治療，リハビリテーションまで「特定の臨床状況のもとで，適切な判断や決断を下せるよう支援する目的で体系的に作成された文書」であり，現在，国際的に標準的な方法とされている「根拠に基づいた医療 Evidence-based Medicine」の手順に則って作成されている（診療ガイドラインの作成の手順 ver. 4.3, 2001）．すべての人が質の高い医療を受けられる，医療関係者の治療の質を向上させるツールとして利用されることが目的であり，あくまでも標準的な指針で，すべての患者に画一的な診療を強制するものではないことに注意すべきである．

　（参考）科学情報はその情報源の種類により，原著論文（一次情報；雑誌論文，学会発表予稿集，研究機関報告書，特許など），二次情報（抄録誌，索引誌など），三次情報（辞書，辞典，全書など）に分けられる．Diabetes Care のような学術雑誌に掲載されている論文は，一次情報にあたる．一次情報の中でも，総説は多くのエビデンス（一般論文や総説など）を要約し解説したものである．このため，総説を読めばその領域の今日の知見を得ることができる．科学情報を evidence として取り扱う場合には，その情報源や情報の質に十分注意が必要である．

Observing the text as a whole

　Look at the following page and think about its PAIL characteristics.　（**PAIL: P** = Purpose 文章の目的，**A** = Audience　文章の対象者，**I** = Information　情報の内容，**L** = Language features　文章の構成形態）

Genre:	Position statement from professional organization　専門家の機関発行の勧告
Purpose:	To state informed opinion and advice of professional community 専門知識に基づく見解や学界からの recommendation を述べる
Audience:	Clinicians and medical team members, including dieticians, and

Information: diabetes patients　臨床医や栄養士を含む医療関係者，糖尿病患者
Specific evidence-based recommendations for nutrition therapy for diabetes　糖尿病患者の食事療法に関する実証研究に基づくrecommendation

Language features: Formal register　フォーマルな表現
Paragraphs　段落構成
Definitions　定義
Large fonts, bold type for section headings　セクションヘディングには，拡大，太字などの字体を使用

Position Statement

Evidence-Based Nutrition Principles and Recommendations for the Treatment and Prevention of Diabetes and Related Complications

American Diabetes Association

INTRODUCTION

Medical nutrition therapy is an integral component of diabetes management and of diabetes self-management education. Yet many misconceptions exist concerning nutrition and diabetes. Moreover, in clinical practice, nutrition recommendations that have little or no supporting evidence have been and are still being given to persons with diabetes. Accordingly, this position statement provides evidence-based principles and recommendations for diabetes medical nutrition therapy. The rationale for this position statement is discussed in the American Diabetes Association technical review "Evidence-Based Nutrition Principles and Recommendations for the Treatment and Prevention of Diabetes and Related Complications," which discusses in detail the published research for each principle and recommendation (1).

Historically, nutrition recommendations for diabetes and related complications were based on scientific knowledge, clinical experience, and expert consensus; however, it was often difficult to discern the level of evidence used to construct the recommendations. To address this problem, the 2002 technical review (1) and this position statement provide principles and recommendations classified according to the level of evidence available using the American Diabetes Association evidence grading system. However, the best available evidence must still take into account individual circumstances, preferences, and cultural and ethnic preferences, and the person with diabetes should be involved in the decision-making process. The goal of evidence-based recommendations is to improve diabetes care by increasing the awareness of clinicians and persons with diabetes about beneficial nutrition therapies.

Because of the complexity of nutrition issues, it is recommended that a registered dietitian, knowledgeable and skilled in implementing nutrition therapy into diabetes management and education, be the team member providing medical nutrition therapy. However, it is essential that all team members be knowledgeable about nutrition therapy and supportive of the person with diabetes who needs to make lifestyle changes.

GOALS OF MEDICAL NUTRITION THERAPY FOR DIABETES

Goals of medical nutrition therapy that apply to all persons with diabetes are as follows:

1. Attain and maintain optimal metabolic outcomes including

- Blood glucose levels in the normal range or as close to normal as is safely possible to prevent or reduce the risk for complications of diabetes.
- A lipid and lipoprotein profile that reduces the risk for macrovascular disease.
- Blood pressure levels that reduce the risk for vascular disease.

2. Prevent and treat the chronic complications of diabetes. Modify nutrient intake and lifestyle as appropriate for the prevention and treatment of obesity, dyslipidemia, cardiovascular disease, hypertension, and nephropathy. 3. Improve health through healthy food choices and physical activity. 4. Address individual nutritional needs taking into consideration personal and cultural preferences and lifestyle while respecting the individual's wishes and willingness to change.

Goals of medical nutrition therapy that apply to specific situations include the following:

1. For youth with type 1 diabetes, to provide adequate energy to ensure normal growth and development, integrate insulin regimens into usual eating and physical activity habits. 2. For youth with type 2 diabetes, to facilitate changes in eating and physical activity habits that reduce insulin resistance and improve metabolic status. 3. For pregnant and lactating women, to provide adequate energy and nutrients needed for optimal outcomes. 4. For older adults, to provide for the nutritional and psychosocial needs of an aging individual. 5. For individuals treated with insulin or insulin secretagogues, to provide self-management education for treatment (and prevention) of hypoglycemia, acute illnesses, and exercise-related blood glucose problems. 6. For individuals at risk for diabetes, to decrease risk by encouraging physical activity and promoting food choices that facilitate moderate weight loss or at least prevent weight gain.

MEDICAL NUTRITION THERAPY FOR TYPE 1 AND TYPE 2 DIABETES

Carbohydrate and diabetes

When referring to common food carbohydrates, the following terms are preferred: sugars, starch, and fiber. Terms such as simple sugars, complex carbohydrates, and fast-acting carbohydrates are not well defined and should be avoided. Studies in healthy subjects and those at risk for type 2 diabetes support the importance of including foods containing carbohydrate particularly from whole grains, fruits, vegetables, and low-fat milk in the diet of people with diabetes.

A number of factors influence glycemic responses to foods, including the amount of carbohydrate, type of sugar (glucose, fructose, sucrose, lactose), nature of the starch (amylose, amylopectin, resistant starch), cooking and food processing (degree of starch gelantinization, particle size, cellular form), and food form, as well as other food components (fat and natural substances that slow digestion-lectins, phytates, tannins, and starch-protein and starch-lipid combinations). Fasting and preprandial glucose concentrations, the severity of glucose intolerance, and the second meal or lente effect of carbohydrate are other factors affecting the glycemic response to foods. However, in persons with type 1 or type 2 diabetes, ingestion of a variety of starches or sucrose, both acutely and for up to 6 weeks, produced no significant differences in glycemic response if the amount of carbohydrate was similar. Studies in controlled settings and studies in free-living subjects produced similar results. Therefore, the total amount of carbohydrate in meals and snacks will be more important than the source or the type.

Studies in subjects with type 1 diabetes show a strong relationship between the premeal insulin dose and the postprandial response to the total carbohydrate content of the meal. Therefore, the premeal insulin doses should be adjusted for the carbohydrate content of the meal. For individuals receiving fixed doses of insulin, day-to-day consistency in the amount of carbohydrate is important.

In persons with type 2 diabetes, on weight maintenance diets, replacing carbohydrate with monounsaturated fat reduces postprandial glycemia and triglyceridemia. However, there is concern that increased fat intake in ad libitum diets may promote weight gain. Therefore, the contributions of carbohydrate and monounsaturated fat to energy intake should be individualized based on nutrition assessment, metabolic profiles, and treatment goals.

Glycemic index.

Although low glycemic index diets may reduce postprandial glycemia, the ability of individuals to maintain these diets long-term (and therefore achieve glycemic benefit) has not been established. The available studies in persons with type 1 diabetes in which low glycemic index diets were compared with high glycemic index diets (study length from 12 days to 6 weeks) do not provide convincing evidence of benefit. In subjects with type 2 diabetes, studies of 2-12 weeks duration comparing low glycemic index and high glycemic index diets report no consistent improvements in HbA1c, fructosamine, or insulin levels. The effects on lipids from low glycemic index diets compared with high glycemic index diets are mixed.

Although it is clear that carbohydrates do have differing glycemic responses, the data reveal no clear trend in outcome benefits. If there are long-term effects on glycemia and lipids, these effects appear to be modest. Moreover, the number of studies is limited, and the design and implementation of several of these studies is subject to criticism.

Fiber.

As for the general population, people with diabetes are encouraged to choose a variety of fiber-containing foods, such as whole grains, fruits, and vegetables because they provide vitamins, minerals, fiber, and other substances important for good health. Early short-term studies using large amounts of fiber in small numbers of subjects with type 1 diabetes suggested a positive effect on glycemia. Recent studies have reported mixed effects on glycemia and lipids. In subjects with type 2 diabetes, it appears that ingestion of very large amounts of fiber are necessary to confer metabolic benefits on glycemic control, hyperinsulinemia, and plasma lipids. It is not clear whether the palatability and the gastro-intestinal side effects of fiber in this amount would be acceptable to most people.

Sweeteners.

The available evidence from clinical studies demonstrates that dietary sucrose does not increase glycemia more than isocaloric amounts of starch. Thus, intake of sucrose and sucrose-containing foods by people with diabetes does not need to be restricted because of concern about aggravating hyperglycemia. Sucrose should be substituted for other carbohydrate sources in the food/meal plan or, if added to the food/meal plan, adequately covered with insulin or other glucose-lowering medication. Additionally, intake of other nutrients ingested with sucrose, such as fat, need to be taken into account.

In subjects with diabetes, fructose produces a lower postprandial response when it replaces sucrose or starch in the diet; however, this benefit is tempered by concern that fructose may adversely effect plasma lipids. Therefore, the use of added fructose as a sweetening agent is not recommended; however, there is no reason to recommend that people with diabetes avoid naturally occurring fructose in fruits, vegetables, and other foods.

Sugar alcohols produce a lower postprandial glucose response than fructose, sucrose, or glucose and have lower available energy values. However, there is no evidence that the amounts likely to be consumed in a meal or day result in a significant reduction in total daily energy intake or improvement in long-term glycemia. The use of sugar alcohols appears to be safe; however, they may cause diarrhea, especially in children.

The Food and Drug Administration has approved four non-nutritive sweeteners for use in the U.S. — saccharin, aspartame, acesulfame potassium, and sucralose. Before being allowed on the market, all underwent rigorous scrutiny and were shown to be safe when consumed by the public, including people with diabetes and during pregnancy.

RESISTANT STARCH

It has been proposed that foods containing naturally occurring resistant starch (cornstarch) or foods modified to contain more resistant starch (high amylose cornstarch) may modify postprandial glycemic response, prevent hypoglycemia, reduce hyperglycemia, and explain differences in the glycemic index of some foods. However, there are no published long-term studies in subjects with diabetes to prove benefit from the use of resistant starch.

Copyright © 2002 American Diabetes Association
From *Diabetes Care*, Vol. 25, 2002; 202-212
Reprinted with permission from the American Diabetes Association

Glossary

age	年齢
aggravate	悪化する
amylose	アミロース（グルコースが直鎖状に重合したデンプン）
clinician	臨床医
cornstarch	コーンスターチ，とうもろこしデンプン
dietitian	栄養士
digest	消化する
discern	見つける，はっきりと認める
dyslipidemia	異常脂質血症（脂質代謝の異常症の総称．高コレステロール血症,高トリグリセリド血症など）
fast	速い
fructose	果糖（グルコースと同じ六単糖でケトンをもつケトヘキソース．吸収の際，グルコースと違いインスリン非依存性であると考えられている）
gelatinization	糊化，アルファ化（デンプンに水と熱を加えることで，デンプンの結晶構造がほどけた状態．米が炊けた状態）
glycemic index	グリセミック指数（等量の炭水化物を含む食品同士を比べ，血糖値の上がり方が早いか遅いかを示す値．グルコース（ブドウ糖）を 100（基準）とする．100 より小さい値の食品ほど血糖値の上昇が緩やかで，食後インスリン値の上昇も緩やかとなることを示す）
hyperglycemia	高血糖（血糖値が高い状態,血糖値が随時 200 mg/100 mL を超える場合に糖尿病と診断される）

hyperinsulinemia	高インスリン血症（血中インスリン濃度が高い状態．常時高い場合，インスリン抵抗性があることを示す）
hypoglycemia	低血糖（血糖値が低い状態，60 mg/100 mL 以下．30 mg/100 mL 以下になると意識レベルが低下し，昏睡状態から死にいたることもある）
individualize	（個々の事情など）に合わせる
ingest	（食物などを）摂取する
intolerance	不耐性（分解できない状態）
isocaloric	等カロリーの
knowledgeable	（〜について）よく知っていて
lactate	乳を分泌する
lactose	ラクトース，乳糖（D-ガラクトースとD-グルコースがβ-1,4 ガラクシド結合した二糖体）
lectins	レクチン類
lente	肉食ぬきの，質素な
lipid	脂質（コレステロール，トリグリセリド，遊離脂肪酸などの総称）
lipoprotein	リポ蛋白（脂質とアポ蛋白が結合したもの，脂質はこの形で血中に存在する）
macrovascular	大血管性の（大動脈などの太い血管のこと）
misconception	誤った考え
monounsaturated	一不飽和の
nephropathy	腎症（腎機能障害のこと．糖尿病性腎症 diabetic nephropathy は神経障害や網膜症に並ぶ，糖尿病の3大合併症のひとつ）
nutritive	栄養の（に関する）
obesity	肥満
palatability	嗜好性，おいしさ
phytate	フィチン酸塩（植物に存在する主要なリンの貯蔵形態．2および3価の金属イオンとキレートをつくる性質をもつため，金属イオンの消化吸収を抑制する）
postprandial	食後の
premeal	食前の
preprandial	食前の，摂食前の
psychosocial	心理社会的な，精神社会的な
rationale	理論的根拠
regimen	（ダイエット・運動などによる），摂生，養生法，食養生
replace	（〜に）取って代わる，（〜を）取り替える
saccharin	サッカリン（人口甘味料）
secretagogue	分泌促進物質
starch	デンプン（植物が光合成により作った栄養源．グルコースが重合した高分子，多糖類，炭水化物）
sucrose	ショ糖，砂糖（ブドウ糖（グルコース）と果糖が結合した2糖体）
sweetener	甘味料（食品に甘みをつけるために用いられるもの．天然品と合成品がある）
tannin	タンニン（植物に存在する収斂性の水溶性物質．蛋白質・アルカロイド・金属イオンと結合して難溶性の塩をつくる）
temper	【他動】和らげる，〜を調節する
triglyceridemia	高トリグリセリド血症（血中の中性脂肪値が高い状態．150 mg/100 mL 以上）

Expanding your vocabulary

Here are some verbs used in the text. Choose the best verb in its grammatically correct form for each of the following sentences. Remember that they are often used in the -ing or -ed form to serve as adjectives.

age	digest	fast	ingest	replace
aggravate	discern	individualize	lactate	temper

1. The data showed that very large amounts of fiber need to be (   ) to have a significant effect.
2. A sweetening agent can be used to (   ) the sugar in food for diabetics.
3. The nurse instructed the patient to (   ) for 12 hours before the blood glucose test.
4. Medicines used for a (   ) mother should not affect the nursing baby.
5. Smoking can (   ) lung diseases.
6. The use of supplements should be (   ) with caution about their overuse.
7. Some foods take a longer time to (   ) than others and remain in the gastrointestinal system for a longer period of time.
8. The doctor could not (   ) any difference in the results from the two test groups in the study.
9. Special medical care is sometimes needed for (   ) individuals.
10. The dietician stated how important it is to (   ) the diet to each person's circumstances.

Reading the text for details

Read the first sentence of each paragraph or the section heading and classify the type of information that can be expected to be presented.

Paragraph

1. Medical nutrition therapy is an integral component of diabetes management and of diabetes self-management education.
2. Historically, nutrition recommendations for diabetes and related complications were based on scientific knowledge, clinical experience, and expert consensus; however, it was often difficult to discern the level of evidence used to construct the recommendations.
3. GOALS OF MEDICAL NUTRITION THERAPY FOR DIABETES
4. MEDICAL NUTRITION THERAPY FOR TYPE 1 AND TYPE 2 DIABETES
5. RESISTANT STARCH

A. What can be done for these types of diseases
B. Background on previous work in this field, the importance of the present work
C. Specific information about food group
D. Background, including importance of this type of therapy
E. What is being aimed for with this kind of therapy

Practicing a text feature

糖尿病患者の食事療法に関する「実証研究に基づく recommendation」について，ここでは，**MEDICAL NUTRITION THERAPY FOR TYPE 1 AND TYPE 2 DIABETES** のセクション中の **Carbohydrate and diabetes** を読み，パラグラフごとに結論を拾い読みしてみましょう．結論は，**Hint expression** をヒントにして見つけましょう．

1. Type2 の糖尿病患者の炭水化物摂取において，重要なことがらを指摘してください．
   Hint expression: Studies in healthy subjects and those at risk for type 2 diabetes support...

2. 対食物血糖反応に影響をおよぼす要因を列挙してください．また，その中でもとりわけ重要な要因を指摘してください．
   Hint expression: A number of factors influence glycemic responses to foods, including... Therefore...

3. Type 1 の糖尿病患者において，食前の insulin 投与量と食事後の炭水化物量に対する応答の間に強い相互関係が見られることから，どのようなことが推奨されていますか？
   Hint expression: Therefore...

4. Type 2 の糖尿病患者において，炭水化物を不飽和脂肪に置き換えることによって，体重増加を抑える療法については，どのようなことが推奨されていますか？
   Hint expression: Therefore...

Saying it yourself   (CD：トラック 13)

A dietician is explaining to a patient with diabetes about the importance of nutrition therapy. Listen for the missing information and then practice the dialogue with a partner.

Dietician: Please have a seat (your partner's name; e.g. Mr. Nakamura, Ms. Yamamoto). I'm (your name; e.g. Yuri Matsumoto, Hideaki Suga). I have been asked to talk to you about how we plan to have nutrition therapy help in the treatment of your (*1.*   ) condition.

Patient: Thank you. The doctor told me that (*2.*   ) can be very effective.

Dietician: Yes. First, let me tell you about what we will be aiming for. There are three important (*3.*   ) that will be our goals. One is to bring your (*4.*   ) to as close to the normal range as possible to prevent complications. Another is to aim for a good lipid profile to reduce the risk of vascular disease.

Patient: I heard that just lowering the (*5.*   ) alone is not the aim.

Dietician: Yes, we want to make sure that you have an adequate amount of "good" cholesterol, or HDL cholesterol.

Patient: I see.

Dietician: The third metabolic outcome we will be aiming for is (*6.*   ).

Patient: It's a bit high as you can see from my medical record.

Dietician: Yes, but if you can lose some weight, that should help lower your blood pressure.

Patient: OK.

Dietician: Some of our other goals will be to prevent any (*7.*   ) of diabetes. Fortunately, you do not seem to have any at present.

Patient: Yes, thank goodness!

Dietician: Well, we must keep it that way. In fact, we will be trying (*8.*   ) with good food and some physical activity.

Patient: That sounds good.

Dietician: Now, in order to help you plan your (9.   ), I need to know something about your personal preferences and (10.   ).

Patient: OK. What would you like to know?

英語あれこれノート

There are many phrases such as the following with Latin words. Sometimes they are used with italic fonts to indicate that they are from a foreign language but many are so frequently used that there is no indication of their foreign origin.

In the above text, "ad libitum" is used.

However, there is concern that increased fat intake in ad libitum diets may promote weight gain.

  ad lib 自由（に）, 任意（に）

Here are some other phrases frequently used in science texts. Can you find examples in your readings?

  in vivo 生体内の
  in vitro 試験管内の
  in situ 生体位の
  in utero 胎内に
  in silico コンピュータ［シリコン］内での ＊試験管内（in vitro）や生体内（in vivo）での実験に対し，コンピュータ利用によるシミュレーション等に基づくもの
  ex vivo 生体外で

英語あれこれノート 解答

Unit1（5ページ）
1. ultraviolet A rays
2. ultraviolet B rays
3. Environmental Protection Agency
4. National Weather Service
5. Sun Protection Factor

Unit3（18ページ）
1 - g
2 - c
3 - d
4 - i
5 - a
6 - b
7 - h
8 - e
9 - f
10 - j

Unit6（41ページ）
1. miso
2. Shiitake
3. sukiyaki
4. Tofu
5. sushi
6. soba
7. Okonomiyaki
8. yakitori
9. ramen

Unit8（55ページ）
1 - D
2 - E
3 - A
4 - B
5 - C

Affixesでみる薬学用語

薬学用語を理解するうえでaffix（接頭辞，接尾辞，語幹）の知識は欠かせません．専門用語は，同じ分野の専門家たちの間で，意味を効率よく伝え合う必要性から生じたものです．一見難しそうに見えますが，affixの知識さえあれば，一語で多くの語義を持つ一般の単語より理解は容易です．特に漢字の知識を持つ日本人の学生にはこの接頭語・接尾語の概念は受け入れやすいはずです．

たとえば，「心電図」といえば，英語では「electrocardiogram」．語順は異なりますが，「心 = cardio, 電 = electro, 図 = gram」となります．このcardio, electro, gramがaffixです．Electroとgramを含む専門用語にはElectroencephalogram「脳電図もしくは脳波図」などがあります．このように初めて出会う専門用語でも単語を構成するaffixがわかれば，大体の見当がつきます．たとえば，「electromyogram」は「筋電図」electrooculogram「眼電図」, electrocorticogram「皮質電図」, electronystagmogram「電気眼振図」です．

Affix	意味	例文
a	without, deficiency, 無，不，非	The strange weather was not an **anomaly**（例外）but an indication of a general trend.
ab	away from, から離れる	The flowers bloomed early this year because of the **abnormally**（異常）warm weather.
abdom	腹部	The belly, or **abdomen**（腹部）, includes the stomach and intestines.
adipo	脂肪	The **adipose**（脂肪）tissue is where energy is stored as fat.
adren	副腎	Corticoid, used as a drug to reduce swelling, is one of the main **adrenocortical**（副腎皮質からの）hormones.
algesi	痛み	He took an **analgesic**（鎮痛剤）to ease the pain from the injury.
an	無（`a-`と同じ；母音の前に置く）	In **anemia**,（貧血）the hemoglobin content of the blood is abnormally low.
angio	血管	**Angiography**（血管造影法）revealed the presence of a clogged blood vessel in the brain.
anti	against, 抗，反対，抑制	**Antineoplastic** agents（抗悪性腫瘍薬）were used to treat the cancer.

Affix	意味	例文
aort	大動脈	Aortitis（大動脈炎）is the inflammation of the main vessel of systemic circulation arising from the heart.
arachno	クモ	A subarachnoid（くも膜下）hemorrhage is due to the rupture of a blood vessel under the cranium.
arterio	動脈	In arteriosclerosis（動脈硬化）, there is abnormal thickening and hardening of the walls of the arteries.
arthr	関節	Arthritis（関節炎）, or inflammation of the joints, can be very painful
bi	two, twice, double, 二, 双, 両	In biology, bilateral（両側）refers to both the right and left sides of the organism.
bio	life, 生命, 生物, 生活, 生体	The biopsy（生検）of the liver showed that the patient had a cancerous tumor.
brachi	上腕	Insert the catheter into the brachial（上腕）vein.
bronchi	気管支	Asthma patients sometimes use bronchodilator（気管支拡張薬）inhalors.
buccal	ほお（頬）	A buccal（ほお）gland（頬腺きょうせん）is a mucous gland located in the membrane lining of the cheeks of mammals.
carcino	癌	Tests of the new food preservative showed that it could be carcinogenic（発がん性の）, causing cancer of the liver.
cardio	心臓	Cardiopathy（心臓病）refers to a diseased condition of the heart.
cephal(o)	頭部, 頭蓋	A cephalopod（頭足動物）is a marine animal, such as cuttlefish and octopus, in which the feet seem to arise from the head.
cerebr(o)	脳,	A cerebral（脳の）infarct , known as a stroke, is caused by a lack of blood supply to the brain.
cervico	首	The bones in the neck region are called the cervical（首の）vertebra（頸椎）.
chole	胆汁	Obesity is an established risk factor for cholelithiasis（胆石症）, or the formation of gall stones in the bile ducts.
cide	殺し	Get the insecticide（殺虫剤）to kill the cockroaches!
circum	円運動, 取り囲む	The circumference（周囲）of a circle is equal to $2\pi r$.
clavi	鎖骨	The subclavian artery（鎖骨下動脈）is proximal part, near the center of the body, of the principal artery in the arm.
clini	医師	He is studying hard to become a clinician（臨床医）because he prefers treating patients to doing research.

Affix	意味	例文
colo	結腸	The woman who had severe abdominal pain was diagnosed as having coloenteritis（全腸炎）.
com, con	共，伴う	The newborn was suffering from a congenital（病気などが生れつきの）heart defect.
conjuncti	結合	The conjunctiva（結膜）is a mucous membrane lining the eyelids.
coron	冠	The coronary（冠状の）arteries（冠状動脈）carry nutrition to the heart.
cortico	皮質	Corticotropin（副腎皮質刺激ホルモン）is a hormonal preparation that has an effect on the adrenal cortex.
cranio	頭蓋	Craniotomy（開頭術）had to be performed on the man who injured his head in the accident.
cut	皮膚	Subcutaneous（皮下）injections place a small amount of fluid through the skin and into the underlying tissue.
cyst	膀胱，胆嚢，嚢胞	The patient got cystitis（膀胱炎）because she did not go to the toilet often enough.
cyto	細胞	A granulocyte（顆粒球）is a white blood cell with a granular cytoplasm.
dactyl	指	Repeated contracting or cramping of a finger or toe is referred to as dactylospasm（指けいれん）.
de	脱，除	The poison was removed by a detoxication（解毒）process.
dent	歯	She went to the dentist（歯科医）to have a decayed wisdom tooth pulled out.
derma	皮膚	The woman suffering from dermatitis（皮膚炎）complained of itchiness of the skin.
di	二，双，複，分離	A dimer（二量体）is a compound formed of two identical molecules.
dis	分離	The man broke his neck in the accident and was disabled（障害のある）for life.
dorsal	背	The dorsal（背面の）fin of the shark is visible when it is swimming near the surface of the ocean.
duodenum	十二指腸	The name of the duodenum（十二指腸）comes from the meaning of twelve fingers to describe its length.
dys	異常，障害，不全，困難	The boy suffered from dyskinesia（運動障害）after the accident and could not walk properly.
emia	血液の状態	Hyperglycemia（高血糖）is a condition in which the blood sugar level is higher than normal.

Affix	意味	例文
encephalo	脳	Japanese encephalitis（脳炎）is a disease causing inflammation of the brain transmitted by a certain mosquito.
endo	内	Endocrinology（内分泌学）is the medicine dealing with glands and their hormones.
entero	腸	Enterorrhagia（腸出血）refers to bleeding from the intestines.
epi	表層，表面	The upper middle portion of the abdomen is called the epigastric（上腹部）area.
equi	等	In chemistry, an equilibrium（化学平衡）is reached when a reversible reaction is balanced so that there is no net change.
erythro	赤血球	Erythrocytes（赤血球）carry the hemoglobin in the blood.
ex(o)	外	An exocrine（外分泌）gland, which as a sweat gland, produces secretions on the outside of the body.
extra	外部，外の	Extrasystole（期外収縮）refers to a disturbance of the heart rhythm in which there is an additional contraction between regular beats.
fetal	胎児の	Pregnant women should not take this drug as it can affect fetal（胎児の）development.
fibro	線維	Fibroblasts（筋膜の線維芽細胞）are large, flat, oval cells which form connective tissues.
fung	カビ	Fungicides（防カビ剤）are used to kill fungi.
gastro	胃	The surgical removal of all or part of the stomach is called gastrectomy（胃切除術）.
gen	原，素	Substances that can cause cancer are called carcinogens（発癌物質）.
genito	生殖器	The genitals（生殖器）refer to the reproductive organs.
gest	消化	A mucous membrane covers the interior of digestive（消化器系）organs.
glyc(o)	糖	Glycolysis（解糖）is a complex series of cellular biochemical reactions that splits glucose, glycogen or other carbohydrates.
gyneco	女性	The medicine dealing with female diseases is called gynecology（女性の）.
hemato	血	Hematuria（血尿）is a pathological condition in which there is blood in the urine.
hepat(o)	肝臓	The drinking of too much alcohol led to his hepatitis（肝炎）.
hexa	六	Hexane（ヘキサン）is a mildly toxic organic compound containing six carbon atoms.

Affix	意味	例文
hidro	汗	A hidrotic（発汗薬）is an agent that can induce sweat.
histo	組織（動植物の）	Tissue structure is investigated by microscopic study in histology（組織学）.
hyper	正常値より上の	Blood pressure that is higher than normal, or hypertension（高血圧）, can be caused by arteriosclerosis.
hypo	（正常値より）下の	A hypodermic（皮下（注射）の）syringe is used to administer medicine into the body.
hystero	子宮	The woman's uterus was removed due to hysterocarcinoma（子宮癌）.
im	非，不	His arm had to be immobilized（固定化した）because the bones were broken.
immuno	免疫	AIDS is the acronym for acquired immunodeficiency（免疫欠損）syndrome.
in	非，不，内部	His inability（無能，不能，できないこと）to do the job properly led to his being fired.
intra	内，内部	We studied the intracellular（細胞内の）organs of a plant using a microscope in botany class.
ischemic	虚血性	In the ischemic（虚血性）state, the amount of inflowing blood decreases extremely.
iso	同，等	An isotherm（等温線）is a line drawn to indicate the same temperature.
kerato	角膜，角質，角化	Nail and hair are composed of keratin（ケラチン）.
kine	運動	Kinesiology（運動療法）is the study of human muscular movements.
lacr	涙	Tears are secreted by the lacrimal（涙液の）gland.
lact(o)	乳汁，乳酸	Yoghurt contains lactobacilli（乳酸菌）which are good for the intestine.
laryng(o)	喉頭	The otorhinolaryngology（耳鼻咽喉科）department treats diseases of the ear, nose and throat.
leuco, leuko	白	The number of leucocytes（白血球）increases greatly when there is infection in the body.
lingu	舌	To administer a drug by the sublingual（舌下の）route, have the patient place the medication under the tongue.
lipo, lipi	脂肪	Lipogenesis（脂質生成）is a process in which fatty acids are produced from smaller molecules, with glucose being the main ingredient.

Affix	意味	例文
lymph(o)	リンパ	In lymphocytosis, there is an abnormally high lymphocyte（リンパ球）count in the blood.
macro	大，巨	Macrovascular（大血管の）diseases are those of the large blood vessels, such as coronary disease.
mammo	乳房	Breast tumors can be detected by mammography（乳房 X 線撮影法）.
melano	黒	A melanoma（黒色腫）is a skin tumor of cells containing dark pigments.
men(o)	月経	Many young women suffer from algomenorrhea（月経痛）once a month.
mening(o)	髄膜，脳脊髄膜	The meninges（髄膜）are three protective membranes surrounding the brain and the spinal cord.
meso	中間，腸間	The mesoderm（中胚葉）is the middle layer of an embryo from which the connective tissue, muscle, bone and blood are formed.
meta	後，中	Metabolism（代謝），from the Greek word for change, is the biosynthesis and breakdown of organic molecules that are essential for life.
micro	小，微小	Bacteria are invisible without a microscope（顕微鏡）.
mis	欠く	The traffic accident caused the miscarriage（流産）of the woman who was in six months pregnant.
mono	単	Mononucleosis（伝染性単核球症）is a condition in which the blood has an excessive number of cells having only one nucleus.
morb	病気	In medical terms, the condition of being diseased is referred to as morbid（病的な，病気の）.
mort	死	The mortality（死亡）rate from traffic accidents decreased after the seat belt law came into effect.
muco	粘液，粘膜	The mucolytic（粘液溶解薬）agent could dissolve or disperse mucus.
multi	多 (= poly, pluri)	She was given multivitamin（マルチビタミン剤）tablets containing a mixture of dietary supplementary substances.
muni	市営の，地方の (= municipal)	The municipal（地方自治体の）waste generated in 2002 in Tokyo reached 52 million tons.
musculo	筋	The inoculation against influenza was given intramuscularly（筋肉注射で）.
myel(o)	骨髄，脊髄	Poliomyelitis（ポリオ，急性灰白髄炎）is a disease that often affected children but can now be prevented with vaccine.

Affix	意味	例文
myo	筋肉	Electromyograms（筋電図）were taken to check for abnormality in the leg muscles.
narc	麻酔，睡眠	Extreme sleepiness can occur due to a disorder called narcolepsy（ナルコレプシー，発作性睡眠）.
nasal	鼻，鼻骨	Nasal sprays（鼻内噴霧）are used to treat stuffed or runny noses.
natal	誕生	That hospital offers good postnatal（出産，出生後の）care after childbirth.
neo	新	Neoplasia（新生組織形成）refers to the growth of new tissue, often the formation of tumors.
nephro	腎	Nephrosis（ネフローゼ）is a degenerative disease of the kidneys.
ness	名詞を示す接尾辞	The feeling of tightness（緊張）in the chest shows that angina can be caused by temporary ischemia.
neur(o)	神経	Neuralgia（神経痛）is a sharp pain along a nerve, especially affecting the face.
non	非，無	Distinguishing between self and non-self（非自己）is important in the immunity mechanism.
obstetri-	助産師	She visits the obstetrician（産科医）regularly because she is in the last trimester of her pregnancy.
oculo	眼	The oculomotor（眼球運動）nerves are responsible for eye movements.
odont(o)	歯	The orthodontist（歯科矯正医）set braces on my teeth to straighten the crooked ones.
ology	〜学	Pathology（病理学）is the branch of medicine that deals with the changes caused by disease.
onco	膨大，腫瘍	The study of cancer is called oncology（腫瘍学）.
ophthalm(o)	眼	For vision problems, consult an ophthalmologist（眼科医）.
opt(o)	視力，視覚	I went to the optometrist（検眼医）to get a new pair of eyeglasses.
oral	口	Brushing your teeth every day is an important part of oral（口腔の）hygiene.
organ(o)	器官，臓器，有機	The formation of organs in an embryo is called organogenesis（器官形成）.
orth(o)	正	She had orthopedic（整形外科）surgery to straighten her nose.
oste(o)	骨	A deficiency of calcium can lead to osteoporosis（骨粗しょう症）.

Affix	意味	例文
oto	耳	Otosclerosis（耳硬化症）is a growth of spongy bone in the inner ear which can cause deafness.
over	〜を超えて	Overdosage（過量投与）means too much of a drug has been taken at one time.
ovi	卵	An oviduct（卵管）is a tube that conducts an egg to the uterus.
pan	すべての, 全体の	People have long searched for a panacea（万能薬）, or a medicine that can cure anything.
path(o)	病気	Scientists tried to identify the pathogen（病原体）of the new disease in order to prevent its spread.
ped	足	My father uses a pedometer（万歩計）check how much exercise he gets during his walks.
pedia	小児, 足	A pediatrician（小児科医）is a physician who specializes in children's diseases.
peri(o)	周囲, 外, 前後	Periodontitis（歯周炎）, resulting from bacterial infection, affects the bone and the gums.
phleb	静脈	The medical term for inflammation of the veins is phlebitis（静脈炎）.
physio	体	Physiology（生理学）is the study of functions and vital processes of living organisms.
pleuro	側腹, 肋骨	Pleurodynia（胸膜痛）refers to a condition of severe pain of the muscles between the ribs.
pneumo	肺	Pneumonia（肺炎）is condition in which the lungs are inflamed and fever develops.
port	運ぶ, 港	Oil is transported（輸送する）by tanker from the Middle East to Japan.
post	後	A high postprandial（食後の）blood glucose level after a meal can sometimes occur is people who are not diabetic.
pre	前	The weather report predicted（予想する）snow for tomorrow.
proof	耐性	A weatherproof（風雨に耐えられる, 全天候型）cover can protect an instrument from bad weather conditions.
psych	精神	Psychoanalysis（精神分析）is used to investigate mental processes and treat disorders of the mind.
pulm	肺	Blood circulation through the lungs is called the pulmonary（肺の）circulation.
radio	放射性	Radiochemistry（放射化学）deals with phenomena in which radiant waves are given off by materials.

Affix	意味	例文
re	再び	We should recycle（再利用）materials to help conserve the natural environment.
renal	腎	The adrenal gland is a suprarenal（副腎の）one located immediately above the kidney.
sacchar	糖	A saccharimeter（サッカリメーター，検糖計）can measure the amount of sugar in a solution.
sarco	肉	A sarcoma（肉腫）is a malignant tumor that begins in the connective tissue.
secrete	分泌	Insulin secreted（分泌される）by the pancreas is the hormone that regulates the blood glucose level.
sinu	曲がりくねった	Sinusitis（副鼻腔炎）is inflammation of the cavities around the nose.
sito	食	Sitology（食品学）is the study of foods, food values and nutrition.
some	体	A microsome（ミクロソーム）is a minute granule in the cytoplasm of an active cell.
somn	睡眠	Talking during sleep is called somniloquence（寝言癖）.
sperm	精子，精液	A spermoblast（精子）is a cell that has a flagellum.
splen	脾臓	A splenectomy（脾臓摘出）had to be performed because a cancerous tumor was detected in the spleen.
stomat(o)	口，口腔	One of the possible causes of stomatitis（口内炎），or inflammation of the mouth mucous membrane, is a lack of vitamin B.
sub	下，下方	The subcellular（細胞内の）mechanism needs to be studied to determine how the drug prevents calcium from entering the cell.
sym	合，癒着，共同	Symbiosis（共生）is a relationship in which two kinds of organisms live together.
syn	合，癒着，共同	He had syndactyly（合指症）with two of his fingers were attached to each other.
thromb(o)	血栓	Thrombosis（血栓症）is a condition in which there is a blood clot in a living blood vessel.
thyro	甲状腺	Dysfunction of the thyroid gland is referred to as thyrosis（甲状腺機能不全）.
tomy	切開	The doctor had to do a tracheotomy（気管切開）to insert an artificial breathing tube because of the severe head and facial injuries.

Affix	意味	例文
tox	毒	Endotoxin（内毒素）is a poisonous substance that remains inside the bacterium until it dies and is broken down.
trans	向こう側へ, 変換	Hair color is a genetically transmitted（(遺伝子)導入された）characteristic.
tri	三	A trimer（三量体）is composed of three identical monomers.
troph	栄養物質	Hypertrophy（肥大）refers to a considerable increase in the size of an organ or tissue.
ultra	超	In ultrafiltration（限外ろ過）, a very dense filter is used for good separation.
un	未, 非, 無	The unauthorized（未許可の）DVD was a pirated version of the new movie.
uni	単一の	The two look like each other because they are uniovular（一卵性の）twins.
ure	尿	A diuretic（利尿の）drug was prescribed to increase urine excretion.
uria	尿	Polyuria（多尿症）refers to an abnormally large volume of urine.
uter	子宮	She went to the gynecologist because she suffered from uterodynia（子宮の痛み）.
vascul(o)	脈管	Vasculitis（脈管炎）is the inflammation of a blood vessel or a lymph vessel.
vaso	血管	Vasodilator（血管拡張を引き起こす）drugs are used to expand the blood vessels.
ven	静脈	Intravenous injection（静脈注射）for rats is difficult because their veins are very narrow.
ventr(o)	腹	Ventrodorsal（腹背の）refers to both the abdominal and back surfaces.
viscer(o)	内臓	The viscera（内臓）are the internal organs of the body, including the heart, lungs, liver and kidneys.
vivi	生	Surgical operations and experiments performed on living animals are referred to as vivisection（生体解剖）.
zoo	動物	Zoonosis（人畜共通感染症）is a disease which can be transmitted from animals to humans.

Vocabulary Index

用語索引

＊発音について

　英単語の発音やアクセントのパターンは，相手に情報を正しく伝えるうえで非常に重要です．特に，カタカナ英語は要注意です．DNA の deoxyribonucleic acid の最初の部分を「ジオクシ」として発音すると，日本人以外の人々にはわかりにくいです．「adenine アデニン」や「guanine グアニン」は理解できますが「thymine チミン」や「cytosine シトシン」は，相手が聞き取りに苦労します．

　また，一音一音の発音以上に大切なのは，アクセントのパターンです．日本人が polymerase「ポリメラーゼ」と言うとき，アクセントが「ラ」に置かれるように聞こえますが，正しい英語のアクセントの位置は二番目の音節です [po LI me reis]．また，[tion] で終わる単語は，後から 2 番目の音節にアクセントが来ます．日本人の話す英語でよく耳にする「IN for mei shun」ではなく「in for MEI shun」になります．

　このように音とアクセントパターンが大体掴めるようにインデックスに簡単な発音表記をヒントとして入れました．発音表記法は色々ありますが，ここでは直感的に理解できるような形をとりました．正確な発音を勉強するには辞書やオンライン辞書（http://www.onelook.com/ のサイトから検索すると，意味や発音記号を呈示するだけでなく，音声機能で実際に発音をしてくれる辞書もあります）を参照してください．

A

a tiny bit	39
abdominal　[ab DO mi nal]	74
abnormality　[ab nor MA li ty]]	60
absenteeism　[ab sen TEE ism]	22
acetaminophen　[a cet a MI no phen]	22
acetylsalicylic acid　[a CET yl sa li CY lic]	22
ad lib	98
additional	16
age	93, 95
aggravate　[AG gra vate]	93, 95
aggravating	23, 25
aggressive　[ag GRES sive]	30
albumen　[al BYU men]	38
albumin　[al BYU men]	38
allergen　[AL ler jen]	38
allergic　[al LER jik]	38
allergist	38
allergy　[AL ler ji]	38
amenable	22
amongst	22
amylose　[AM a lous]	93
analgesia　[an al GE zi a]	22
analgesic　[an al GE zik]	23
anaphylactic　[a na fi LAK tik]	38
anaphylaxis　[a na fi LAK sis]	38, 39
aneurysm　[AN yu ri zim]	22
angina　[an JAI na]	82
annual	16
anomaly　[a NOM a lee]	60
antis　[AN tiz]	8
appendicitis　[ap pen di SI tis]	19
appliance　[ap PLI ance]	31
aromatic　[a ro MAT ic]	59
arterial　[ar TE ri al]	8, 67, 82
arteries　[AR te riz]	9, 68
arthritis　[ar THRI tis]	19
ASEAN　[A se an]	5
atherosclerosis　[ATH e ro scle RO sis]	82, 83
atrium　[AY tri um]	67

auspices   [AUS pi ces]   30

B

baked goods   39
beef   55
biometrics   [bi o MET rics]   15
biphenyl   [bai PHEN il]   59, 64
bleached   [BLEACH d]   60
blurry   15
bracketing   67
brain   23
breathing   [BREETH ing]   39
brim   3
broad spectrum sunscreen   3
buildup   74
bulky   30
byproduct   [BAI pro duct]   59

C

caffeine withdrawal   22
calf   55
canopy   [KA no pi]   3
capillary   [KAP il la ri]   67, 68
carcinogen   [kar SIN o jen]   59
carcinogenic   [KAR sin o JEN ik]   59
carcinogenicity   [KAR sin o je NI ci ti]   59
cardiovascular   [KAR di o VAS kyu lar]
   9, 74, 82, 83
casein   [KAY seen]   38
caseinate   [KAY see nate]   38
cataract   [KAT a ract]   3
causative   [KAW za tive]   82
cephalalgia/cephalgia/cephalea   [se fal AL gi a]   22
cerebral   [se RE bral]   23
cessation   [se SA shun]   82
chicken   55
chlorinate   [KLOr I nate]   59
cholesterol synthesis inhibitor   [ko LES te rol]   82
circumference   [sur KUM frens]   74
clinical   16, 83
clinician   [kli NI shun]   93
clot   8
clotting   9
cold sweat   74
combustible   [kom BUS ti bl]   30
complicate   25
complication   45
concerned (with symptoms)   [kon SERND]   23
confusion   [kon FYU zhun]   74
congener   [KON je ner]   59

congenital   [kon JEN i tal]   59
conjunctival   [KON junk TI val]   16
conjunctivitis   [kon junk ti VI tus]   19
contagious   [kon TAI jus]   53
contaminant   [kon TAMI nant]   60
coordination   31
coplanar/planar   [KO play ner]   59
cornea   [KOR ni a]   15
corneal   [KOR ni al]   16
cornstarch   93
coronary   [KO ro na ri]   82, 83
correlate   [KOR re late]   74
corticosteroid   [kor ti co STE roid]   15
cow   55
cramp   38
criteria   74
cystitis   [sis TAI tis]   19
cytochrome P450   [SAI to krom pi four fifty]   59, 64

D

dehydrated   [di HAI drei ted]   23, 25
delirium   [di LI ri um]   45
deoxygenated blood   [di OXY je nei ted]   67, 68
deoxygenation   [di oxy je NEI shun]   67
dermatitis   [der ma TAI tis]   19
designate   [DE zig nate]   30
dibenzofuran   [DAI ben zo FU ran]   59, 64
dietary   [DAI e te ri]   82
dietitian   [dai e TI shan]   93
digest   [dai JEST]   93, 95
digestive   [dai JES tiv]   82
dioxin   [dai OX in]   60, 62
discern   [dis CERN]   93, 95
discomfort   [dis COM fort]   74
dishes   39
disinfect   [dis in FECT]   15
dizziness   [DIZ i nes]   74
domesticated   [do MES ti kai ted]   52
dry   23
dumping ground   34
dustbin   34
dustcart   34
dyslipidemia   [dis li pi DE mi a]   93

E

elevate   [E le vait]   82
emulsification   [e mul si fi KAI shun]   82
enacted   [en AK ted]   30
encephalitis   [en se fa LAI tis]   19, 22
enchilada   [en shi LA da]   38

endocrine [EN do krin]	60
endogenous [en DO ji nus]	82
endometriosis [en do me tri O sis]	60
EPA	5
epidemiological [e pe di mi o LO ji kul]	9
epidemologic [e pe di mi o LO jik]	60
equivalency [e KWI ve len si]	60
ex vivo [eks VI vo]	98
excretion [eks KRE shun]	53
exogenous [eks ZA je nus]	82
expel [eks PEL]	39
explain	25
extracellular [eks tra SEL lu lar]	67
extrude [eks TRUD]	39
eyestrain	22

F

fast	93, 95
feasibility [fe za BI li ty]	82
feces [FE ses]	52, 53
feverfew [FEV er fyu]	22
feverish [FEV er ish]	9
fibric acid derivative [FAI brik a sid de RIV a tiv]	82
fibrinolysis [fai bri NO li sis]	8
fibroblast [FAI bro blast]	82
fibrogen [FAI bro jen]	8
fibrous [FAI brus]	82
fructose [FRUK tos]	93
fungal [FUN gul]	16

G

garbage can [GAR bej kan]	34
garbage incinerating facility [GAR bej in SIN a rei ting fa SI li ti]	34
garbage truck	34
gastritis [gas TRI tis]	19
gastrointestinal [gas tro in TES ti nl]	67, 82
gelatinization [je la ti ni ZAI shun]	93
generalize [JE ne ra laiz]	82
glycemic index [GLAI se mik]	93
goods	39

H

hallucination [hal lu si NAI shun]	45
HDL	8
headache [HED aik]	23
healthcare	22
hemagglutinin [he ma GLU ti nin]	52
hepatitis [he pa TAI tis]	19
hepatocyte [he PA to sait]	82
herbal [HUR bl]	22
herbicide [HUR be side]	60
hexa- [HEK sa]	60
high density lipoprotein [li po PRO teen]	82
hoarseness	39
hyperglycemia [hai per glai SE mi a]	74, 93
hyperinsulinemia [hai per in su li NE mi a]	94
hyperlipidemia [hai per li pi DE mi a]	74
hypertension [HAI per ten shun]	74
hypoglycemia [hai po glai SE mi a]	94

I, J

ibuprofen [AI byu PRO fen]	22
immunocompromised [im myu no KOM pro mizd]	15
immunodeficiency [im myu no de FI shun si]	15
immunologic [im myu no LO jik]	60
immunologist [im myu NO lo jist]	39
impaired [im PEARD]	60
in silico [in SIL i ko]	98
in situ [in SIT u]	98
in utero [in UT e ro]	98
in vitro [in VIT ro]	98
in vivo [in VIV o]	98
inactivity [in ak TIV i ty]	74
incinerated [in SIN e rai ted]	60
individualize [in di VI zu a laiz]	94, 95
industrialize [in DUS tri a laiz]	82
inexplicable [in ex PLI ka bl]	9
infarction [in FARK shun]	82
influenza [in flu EN za]	53
ingest [in JEST]	60, 94, 95
initiate [i NI shi ate]	15
insomnia [in SOM ni a]	9
insulate [IN su lait]	60
intestine [in TES tin]	53
intolerance [in TO le rens]	94
intrauterine [in tra YU te rin]	60
ion-exchange resin [ai on eks chainj RE zin]	82
ischaemia [is KE mi a]	9
ischaemic [is KE mik]	8
isocaloric [ai so KA lo rik]	94
itch [ICH]	39
itchy [ICH i]	39
JAMA [JA ma]	5

K

keratitis [ke ra TAI tis]	15
kinetics [ki NE tics]	82
knowledgeable [NO le ja bl]	94

L

lactalbumin [lact AL bu min]		39
lactate [LAC teit]		94, 95
lactoglobulin [lac to GLO bu lin]		39
lactose [LAC tos]		94
lactulose [LAC tu los]		39
lamb		55
landfill		60
LDL		8
lecithin [LE si thin]		39
lectin [LEC tin]		94
lente [LEN te]		94
liberally [LI be ra li]		3
lightheadedness		74
lint		15
lipid [LI pid]		82, 94
lipoprotein [li po PRO teen]		74, 82, 83, 94
longevity [lon JE vi ti]		9
loss of coordination		74
low density lipoprotein		82
lumen [LU men]		83
lymphocytic [lim pho SI tik]		60
lymphoma [lim PHO ma]		60

M

macrovascular [ma kro VAS cu lar]		94
marzipan [MART zi pan]		39
medical		16
medication		15
meninges [me NIN jez]		22
meningitis [me nin JAI tis]		22
menopause [MEN o paz]		8
menstruation [men STRA shun]		22
meringue [me RANG]		39
metabolic [me ta BO lik]		74, 83
MEXT		5
microbial [mai KRO bi al]		16
midday [MID day]		3
migraine [MAI grain]		23
misconception [mis kon SEP shun]		94
moderation [mo de RAI shun]		9
monounsaturated [mo no un SAT u rei ted]		94
mortality rate [mor TA li ti reit]		53
muggy [MUG gi]		8
multipurpose		15
municipal [myu NI si pl]		30
municipality [myu ni ci PA lity]		30
myocardial [my o CAR di al]		83

N

narcotic [nar KO tik]		23
nasal		53
nausea [NAW ze a]		74
neomycin [ne o MAI sin]		83
nephritis [ne FRAI tis]		19
nephropathy [ne FRO pa thi]		94
neuraminidase [nur a MI ni deis]		53
neurological [nyu ro LOJ i kul]		60
neuropathy [nyu RO pa thi]		60
neuropsychiatric [nyu ro sai ki A trik]		45
nicotinic acid [ni ko ti nik A sid]		83
nomenclature [NO men kla tur]		60
noncombustible [non kum BUS ti bl]		30
northeasterly		8
notification		15
nougat [NU gut]		39
NSAID (nonsteroidal anti-inflammatory drug) [EN seid]		22
nullify [NUL li fi]		8
numbness [NUM ness]		74
nutrient [NYU tri ent]		67
nutritive [NYU tri tiv]		94
NWS		5

O

obesity [o BE si ti]		74, 94
ocular [O kyu lar]		15
organochlorine [or ga no KLO reen]		60
ortho- [OR tho]		60, 64
outdoors		3
outgrow		39
overexposure		3
overweight		74
oxygenated blood [OK si je nei ted blud]		67, 68
oxygenation [ok si je NEI shun]		67

P

painkiller		22
palatability [pa la ta BI li ti]		94
pandemic [pan DE mik]		45
paracetamol [pa ra CE ta mol]		22
partial [PAR shul]		16
pathogenic [pa tho JE nik]		53
pathophysiology [pa tho fi si O lo gee]		23
peanut butter		39
pecan [pe KAAN]		39
penta- [PEN ta]		60
pernicious [per NI sh us]		8
pharmacy [FAR ma ci]		31

phosphate [FOS fayt]	39
physiology (of abnormal states) [fi si O lo gee]	23
phytate	94
pig	55
pneumonia [nyu MO ni a]	53
pork	55
porphyria [por FE ri a]	60
portal [POR tul]	67, 68
postprandial [post PRAN de ul]	94
poultry [POL tree]	55
precipitate [pre CI pi teit]	22
precursor [pre KUR sur]	83
premeal	94
preprandial [pre PRAN de ul]	94
prescribe [pre SKRIB]	15
preventative [pre VEN ta tiv]	23
preventive [pre VEN tiv]	23
primate [PRI meit]	83
probucol [PRO bu kol]	83
professional [pro FES shun al]	16
prone to [proun tu]	3
psychosocial [sai co SO shul]	94
pulmonary [PUL mo na ri]	67, 68

R

radiological [rei di o LO ji kul]	16
rationale [ra sho NAAL]	94
reabsorb [RE ab zorb]	83
reapply [RE ap pli]	3
rebound [RE bound]	22
receptor [re SEP tor]	60
rechargeable [re CHARG a bul]	30
recommended [re kom MEN ded]	25
redness [RED ness]	15
regenerate [re JEN e reit]	83
regimen [RE ji men]	16, 94
rennet [REN net]	39
replace [re PLAIS]	94, 95
report [re PORT]	45
require	16
resin [RE zin]	83
restaurant	39
retardation	60
reviewer	45
rinse	16
rubbish bag	34
ruffled	53
runny	39

S

saccharin [SAK a rin]	94
saliva [sa LAI va]	53
sarcoma [sar KO ma]	60
scalp [skalp]	22, 39
scavenger [SKA ven jer]	83
secretagogue [se KREET a gog]	94
secrete [se KREET]	83
sheep	55
shellfish	39
shortness (of breath)	74
simple	23
sinusitis [si nyu SAI tis]	22
sitosterol [sai TOS te rol]	83
sizable [SAIZ a bl]	60
sneeze	39
SPF	4, 5
starch	94
steroid [STE roid]	83
stickiness	8
stockpile	45
stomatitis [sto ma TAI tis]	19
stuffy	39
substituted [SUB sti tu ted]	60
subtype [SUB type]	53
sucrose [SU kros]	94
sunbed	3
sunglasses	3
sunlamps	3
sunscreen	3
sweetener	94
symptomatic [symp to MA tik]	23
synthesize [SYN the saiz]	83
syringe [su RINJ]	30
systemic [sis TE mik]	16, 67, 68

T

tannin [TAN nin]	94
tanning parlor	3
teetotaller [tee TO ta ler]	8
temper [TEM per]	94, 95
TEPCO [TEP ko]	5
threatening	25, 30
throat	39
throat tightness	39
times2	8
tingling [TIN gling]	39
toddler	39
topical [TOP i kul]	16

toxicity　[tok SI si ti]	60
traction　[TRAK shun]	22
transitional	67
transplantation	16
trash	60
trash bag	34
tri-　[trai]	60, 64
triglyceride　[trai GLI se raid]	74
triglyceridemia　[trai gli se ri DE mi a]	94
Tylenol®　[TAI le nol]	22

U

unclear	23
uncomplicated	23, 25
undetected	53
unexplained	23, 25
unintentional	60
universally	67
unprotected	3
unsubstituted	60
utilization	30
utilize	83
UV	3
UV Index	3
UVA	5
UVB	5

V

vascular　[VAS kyu lar]	67
vasoconstrictor　[va so con STRIK tor]	22
veal	55
vein	68
vendor	31
virulence　[VI ru lens]	53
vomit	39

W

waterfowl	53
waterproof	3
weakness	74
wheeze　[weez]	39
workaholic	8
worsening	23

著者紹介

野口　ジュディー（Ph.D.）
2001 年　The University of Birmingham, School of English 研究科修了
現　在　神戸学院大学グローバル・コミュニケーション学部教授（学部長）
　　　　大阪大学工学研究科　非常勤講師
　　　　大阪大学医学研究科　非常勤講師
　　　　武庫川女子大学薬学部　非常勤講師

神前　陽子（教育博士）
2006 年　テンプル大学大学院英語教授法研究科修了
現　在　武庫川女子大学薬学部　非常勤講師
　　　　神戸大学大学院理学研究科　非常勤講師
　　　　テンプル大学応用言語学博士課程　非常勤講師
　　　　大阪薬科大学　非常勤講師

籠田　智美（薬学博士）
1990 年　武庫川女子大学大学院薬学研究科修了
現　在　武庫川女子大学薬学部　准教授

山口　秀明（農学博士）
1995 年　名古屋大学大学院農学研究科満期退学
現　在　名城大学農学部　教授

NDC491　　124p　　26cm

入門薬学英語

2007 年 3 月 20 日　第 1 刷発行
2016 年 2 月 20 日　第 9 刷発行

著　者　野口ジュディー・神前陽子・籠田智美・山口秀明
発行者　鈴木　哲
発行所　株式会社　講談社
　　　　〒 112-8001　東京都文京区音羽 2-12-21
　　　　　販売　(03) 5395-4415
　　　　　業務　(03) 5395-3615
編　集　株式会社　講談社サイエンティフィク
　　　　代表　矢吹俊吉
　　　　〒 162-0825　東京都新宿区神楽坂 2-14　ノービィビル
　　　　　編集　(03) 3235-3701
ＤＴＰ　株式会社エヌ・オフィス
印刷所　株式会社平河工業社
製本所　株式会社国宝社

落丁本・乱丁本は購入書店名を明記のうえ，講談社業務宛にお送りください．送料小社負担にてお取替えします．なお，この本の内容についてのお問い合わせは，講談社サイエンティフィク宛にお願いいたします．価格はカバーに表示してあります．

© J. Noguchi, Y. Kozaki, S. Kagota and H. Yamaguchi, 2007

本書のコピー，スキャン，デジタル化等の無断複製は著作権法上での例外を除き禁じられています．本書を代行業者等の第三者に依頼してスキャンやデジタル化することはたとえ個人や家庭内の利用でも著作権法違反です．

JCOPY　〈(社) 出版者著作権管理機構委託出版物〉

複写される場合は，その都度事前に (社) 出版者著作権管理機構（電話 03-3513-6969，FAX 03-3513-6979，e-mail: info@jcopy.or.jp）の許諾を得てください．

Printed in Japan

ISBN978-4-06-155611-9

講談社の自然科学書

はじめての薬学英語 CD付き	野口ジュディーほか／著	価格 2,500円
入門薬学英語 CD付	野口ジュディーほか／著	価格 2,800円
医療薬学英語	野口ジュディーほか／著	本体 3,000円
ニュースで読む 医療英語 CD付き	川越栄子ほか／編著	本体 2,800円
医療従事者のための医学英語入門	清水雅子／著	本体 2,500円
チーム医療のためのメディカル英語 基本表現100	木久代・小澤淑子／編著　矢田 公／著	本体 2,400円
耳から学ぶ 楽しいナース英語 CD付	中西睦子／監修　野口ジュディーほか／著	本体 3,400円
Judy先生の耳から学ぶ科学英語 CD付き	野口ジュディー／著	本体 3,400円
Judy先生の英語科学論文の書き方 増補改訂版	野口ジュディーほか／著	本体 3,000円
Judy先生の成功する理系英語プレゼンテーション CD付き	野口ジュディーほか／著	価格 2,800円
科学者のための英文手紙・メール文例集 CD-ROM付き	阪口玄二・逢坂 昭／著	価格 3,500円
医学・薬学系のための基礎生物学	八杉貞雄／編著	本体 3,800円
医歯薬系のための生物学	小林 賢／編著	本体 4,400円
薬剤師のためのコミュニケーションスキルアップ	井手口直子／編著	本体 2,800円
わかりやすい薬学系の数学入門	都築 稔／編	本体 2,800円
わかりやすい薬学系の化学入門	小林 賢ほか／編　杉田一郎ほか著	本体 2,800円
わかりやすい薬学系の統計学入門	小林 賢ほか／編　井上俊夫ほか著	本体 2,800円
わかりやすい薬学系の物理学入門	小林 賢ほか／編　安西和紀ほか著	本体 2,800円
スタートアップ 服薬指導	大井一弥／編著	本体 2,400円
ビタミンの新栄養学	柴田克己・福渡 努／編	本体 4,800円
がんばろう薬剤師	村徳人／著	本体 1,800円
今日から使える漢方薬のてびき	入江祥史・坂井由美／著	本体 2,200円
スタートアップ がん薬物治療	大井一弥／編著	本体 2,900円
医学部編入への生命科学演習	松野 彰／監修　井出冬章／著　河合塾KALS／協力	本体 4,300円
医学部編入への英語演習	河合塾KALS／監修　土田 治／著	本体 4,000円
大学1年生の なっとく！生物学	田村隆明／著	本体 2,300円
いちばんやさしい生化学	坂本順司／著	本体 2,200円
ひとりでマスターする生化学	亀井碩哉／著	本体 3,800円
カラー図解 生化学ノート	森 誠／著	本体 2,200円
よくわかる分子生物学・細胞生物学実験 原理＆実験の組み立て方	佐々木博己／編・著	本体 3,400円

※表示価格は本体価格（税別）です。消費税が別に加算されます。　「2016年2月現在」

講談社サイエンティフィク　http://www.kspub.co.jp/